Fast Facts

Fast Facts:
Non-Small-Cell
Lung Cancer

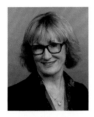

Mary O'Brien MD FRCP
Consultant Medical Oncologist
The Royal Marsden NHS Foundation Trust
London, UK

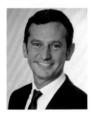

Benjamin Besse MD PhD
Thoracic Cancer Unit, Head
Department of Cancer Medicine
Gustave Roussy
Villejuif, France

Declaration of Independence
This book is as balanced and as practical as we can make it.
Ideas for improvement are always welcome: feedback@fastfacts.com

✝ HEALTH PRESS

Fast Facts: Non-Small-Cell Lung Cancer
First published September 2016
Text © 2016 Mary O'Brien, Benjamin Besse

© 2016 in this edition Health Press Limited
Health Press Limited, Elizabeth House, Queen Street, Abingdon,
Oxford OX14 3LN, UK
Tel: +44 (0)1235 523233

Book orders can be placed by telephone or via the website.
For regional distributors or to order via the website, please go to:
fastfacts.com
For telephone orders, please call +44 (0)1752 202301.

Fast Facts is a trademark of Health Press Limited.

A CIP record for this title is available from the British Library.

ISBN 978-1-910797-19-8

O'Brien M (Mary)
Fast Facts: Non-Small-Cell Lung Cancer/
Mary O'Brien, Benjamin Besse

Cover image: colored chest X-ray showing lung cancer in frontal view.

Medical illustrations by Annamaria Dutto, Withernsea, UK.
Typesetting by Thomas Bohm, User Design, Illustration and Typesetting, UK.
Printed in the UK with Xpedient Print.

Introduction

Lung cancer is the commonest preventable cancer of the 21st century. As smoking cessation initiatives take effect its incidence should decrease, but we are still facing a large burden of disease for at least the next 30 years, with non-small-cell lung cancer (NSCLC) accounting for 80% of the load.

This insightful guide is designed to bring you up to speed with the latest developments. It provides a concise, practical overview of new targeted therapies, the latest CT-based screening approaches and the use of stereotactic radiation for early-stage tumors, together with the latest revisions to the lung cancer classification for small biopsies and cytology specimens and lung cancer TNM staging system.

While early detection strategies should increase identification of patients with early-stage disease – who can usually be cured with a combination of surgery, chemotherapy and radiotherapy – most patients with NSCLC still present with locally advanced or metastatic disease. Proposed changes to the TNM classification system will improve the accuracy of staging in these individuals, and we predict that up to 50% of patients with advanced NSCLC will benefit from some form of targeted treatment over the next 5 years. Furthermore, modulation of the immune system and the subsequent opportunities for personalized treatment will have a profound positive effect on the natural history of NSCLC.

Fast Facts: Non-Small-Cell Lung Cancer is important reading for all health professionals and medical trainees working in this fast-moving area.

David Walder MBBS BSc MRCP(UK), *Department of Medical Oncology, The Royal Marsden NHS Foundation Trust, London, UK*

Lung cancer is the leading cause of cancer death in both men and women in the USA and worldwide.[1,2] In Europe, lung cancer in women is set to overtake breast cancer as the leading cause of cancer-related mortality.[3] Non-small-cell lung cancer (NSCLC), which includes adenocarcinoma, squamous cell carcinoma and large cell carcinoma, accounts for approximately 80–85% of all lung cancers. Small-cell lung cancer (SCLC) accounts for the other 15%.

Risk factors

Tobacco smoke is the most important cause of lung cancer. Close to 90% of all lung cancers are attributable to cigarette smoke, of which a small proportion are due to second-hand smoke.[1] The number of cigarettes smoked, but more importantly the length of time that patients have smoked for, is proportional to the risk of developing lung cancer. Evidence from the landmark 1964 Surgeon General's report estimated that an average male smoker had a nine- to tenfold increased risk of developing lung cancer compared with a 'never smoker'. For heavy smokers (more than 25 cigarettes per day) the risk is at least 20-fold.[4]

Ex-smokers who have quit for more than 15 years show an 80–90% reduction in their risk of lung cancer compared with persistent smokers. The risk reduces by 50% in the first decade and continues to decrease the longer the duration of abstinence.[1] Approximately 1 in 9 smokers develop lung cancer. Individual susceptibility to developing lung cancer is affected by genetic predisposition and other environmental factors.

Environmental factors. Many occupational exposures increase the risk of developing lung cancer (Table 1.1).[5] These are likely to be underestimated because of lack of detailed occupational histories and the synergistic effect of tobacco smoke with many occupational

TABLE 1.1

Common occupational agents associated with increased risk of lung cancer as classified by the International Agency for Research on Cancer (IARC)

Agent	Frequent sources of exposure
Asbestos	Electrical insulation, shipyard work, brakes, textile industry, mining, plumbing
Beryllium and beryllium oxide	Nuclear technology, electronics
Arsenic, arsenic compounds	Agriculture, glass manufacturing
Cadmium	Batteries, pigments
Nickel compounds	Mining, milling, stainless steel manufacturing
Silica dust and quartz	Ceramics, sandblasting, mining
Paints and solvents	Decorators, chemists
Chromium	Production of electroplating
Chloromethyl ether	Plastic manufacturing

carcinogens. Asbestos fiber exposure is the most common occupational cause of NSCLC (usually adenocarcinoma as well as mesothelioma), and the effect is potentiated in smokers.

High levels of household radon, due to a naturally occurring radioactive gas (radon 222) formed from the breakdown of uranium in soil and rock, increases the incidence of lung cancer and lung cancer deaths. Domestic radon levels vary widely within and between countries. In Europe, lower levels are seen in countries with predominantly sedimentary soil types such as the UK, Germany and the Netherlands compared with areas with old granite soil such as Austria, the Czech Republic and Finland.

Family history and genetics. Patients with a first-degree relative with lung cancer have a 50% increased risk of developing lung cancer. The effect is greatest in those with a sibling with lung cancer and is seen regardless of smoking status.

Genome-wide association studies have shown that a major susceptibility locus on chromosome 6q (6q23–25p) is associated with increased lung cancer risk.[6] Smoking increases the risk further. Multiple studies have found another susceptible marker on chromosome 15. Three genes in this region code for subunits of the nicotinic acetylcholine receptor. It is postulated that mutations in these genes influence lung cancer risk by increasing vulnerability to nicotine addiction. Targeting genetically high-risk individuals for intensive smoking cessation and screening programs may be the focus for future lung cancer prevention strategies.

Underlying disease. Chronic obstructive pulmonary disease (COPD) is associated with lung cancer risk.[7] Although tobacco smoke is a common etiologic factor, airway obstruction is an independent risk factor and may provide a potential pathogenic explanation. Idiopathic pulmonary fibrosis (IPF) is also associated with a sevenfold increase in lung cancer risk.[8] A meta-analysis of diabetic patients has shown an increased lung cancer risk, especially in women.[9]

Previous malignancy. Lung cancer is frequently seen in survivors of previous malignancies, particularly other smoking-related malignancies. Cohort studies have shown increased risk following non-Hodgkin's lymphoma, testicular cancer, uterine sarcomas and head and neck cancers.[10] Patients who have had radiation therapy for thoracic malignancies (e.g. lymphomas) are at increased risk of lung cancer; smoking further increases the risk. In patients with breast cancer who have never smoked, postmastectomy radiotherapy is associated with an almost twofold increase in lung cancer risk in the ipsilateral lung but not the contralateral lung.[11]

Impaired immunity. Patients with HIV infection have consistently been shown to have increased rates of lung cancer and are diagnosed at an earlier age. Although the prevalence of cigarette smoking within the HIV-positive population is higher than the general population, a meta-analysis revealed a 2.5-fold increased risk of developing lung cancer in HIV-positive patients independent of smoking status.[12]

Lifestyle factors. A systematic review by the World Cancer Research Fund found 'probable' evidence that greater levels of fruit, and to a lesser extent vegetable consumption, are inversely associated with lung cancer risk.[13] Disappointingly, a large randomized double-blind placebo-controlled trial of daily supplementation with vitamin A and β-carotene was stopped prematurely as there was clear evidence of no benefit and substantial evidence of harm.[14]

A recent Cochrane review found no evidence that vitamin D supplementation had any effect on lung cancer risk.[15] There is only weak evidence to suggest that high physical activity can reduce the risk of lung cancer. The evidence for a protective effect of acetylsalicylic acid (ASA; aspirin) on lung cancer risk is inconsistent and limited to case control studies.

Screening

In around 70% of cases, patients with lung cancer present to secondary care with symptomatic, advanced, incurable disease. Although mass screening of high-risk asymptomatic patients has the potential to detect disease at an earlier stage, randomized trials using chest X-ray (CXR) have not shown a reduction in lung-cancer mortality.[16] More recently, trials have focused on the use of low-dose computed tomography (LDCT). The largest of these, the US-based National Lung Screening Trial (NLST), in which 53 454 current and former smokers (> 30 pack-years) aged 55–74 years were randomized to LDCT or CXR, showed a 20% relative reduction in lung cancer-related mortality and a 6.7% reduction in all-cause mortality in patients screened by LDCT.[17]

Challenges to lung cancer screening are concerns over false positives, complications during diagnostic work-up, patient anxiety and screening cost.

The large Dutch–Belgian NELSON trial randomized 15 882 lower-risk participants (age 50–75 years, 15 pack-years, smoking within 10 years of trial) to annual LDCT or a control arm. The controls did not undergo CXR screening, unlike the controls in the NLST. The NELSON trial benefited from the use of volumetric analysis and volume doubling time assessment to determine interval growth of indeterminate pulmonary nodules. Consequently, there were far fewer false-positive screens and invasive diagnostic tests in the NELSON trial than in the NLST.[18] Survival data are awaited.

Advances in lung cancer screening are likely to involve refining the target population by identifying high-risk groups using risk prediction models such as the Liverpool Lung Project (LLP$_{v2}$) risk model to identify people with a 5% or greater 5-year risk of developing lung cancer.[19]

The United States Preventative Services Task Force supports the screening of healthy adults between 55 and 80 years of age with a minimum of 30 pack-years smoking history and who have smoked within the previous 15 years. The European Respiratory Society and the European Society of Radiology agree, but this is currently not funded in most European countries.[20]

Solitary peripheral nodules

Pulmonary nodules are small (< 3 cm diameter) focal opacities identified on imaging. Diagnostic algorithms depend on the size and radiological appearance of the nodule (Table 1.2; Figures 1.1 and 1.2) and the pre-test probability of malignancy (Figure 1.3). Verified risk assessment tools (e.g. the Brock model) have been shown to be more accurate than clinician assessment at predicting risk of malignancy.

Unless there are obvious features of benign disease, nodules found on CT should be compared for interval growth. A semi-automated software program allows the calculation of nodule volume doubling time to stratify the risk of malignancy.

TABLE 1.2

Definition and nomenclature of pulmonary nodules

Solid nodule	Focal rounded ≤ 3 cm opacity surrounded mostly by aerated lung
Sub-solid nodule	Part-solid or pure ground glass ≤ 3 cm opacity
Part-solid nodule	Focal opacity containing both solid and ground glass components (Figure 1.1)
Pure ground glass nodule (pGGN)	Focal opacity that does not completely obscure the vascular pattern (Figure 1.2)

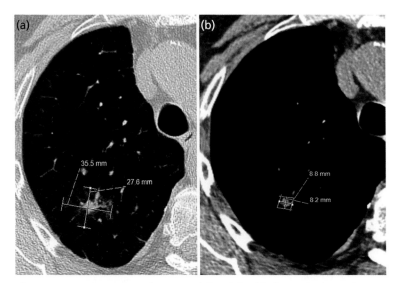

Figure 1.1 Measurement of a part-solid nodule. (a) The entire lesion is visible on the lung window, but (b) only the solid component can be measured on the mediastinal window.

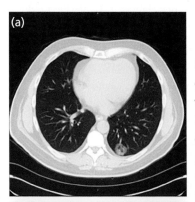

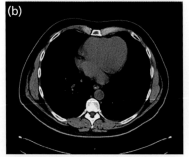

Figure 1.2 CT scan of a pure ground glass nodule (pGGN). (a) On the lung window, the pGGN is visible in the left lower lobe of the lung. (b) On the mediastinal window, the pGGN is not visible. This technique can be used to help identify part-solid nodules. Reproduced from *Journal of Community Hospital Internal Medicine Perspectives* 2014;4:24562. http://dx.doi.org/10.3402/jchimp. v4.24562, last accessed 11 August 2016.

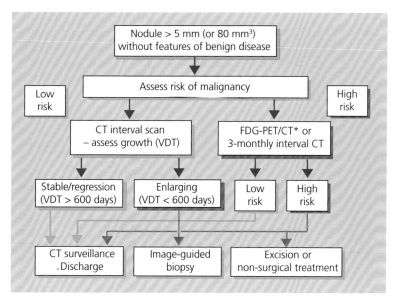

Figure 1.3 Diagnosis of a pulmonary nodule. Sub-solid nodules may not be fludeoxyglucose (FDG) avid; therefore management decisions will depend on risk stratification after interval imaging. —— High risk (> 10%) of malignancy. Treatment decision should take into account individual risk profile and patient preference. —— Low risk (< 10%) of malignancy. Surveillance for 1–4 years depends on size and morphological factors. *Use PET where nodule is larger than local PET-CT detection threshold. FDG-PET/CT, fludeoxyglucose positron emission tomography/computed tomography; VDT, volume doubling time. Adapted from British Thoracic Society guidelines for the investigation and management of pulmonary nodules; local guidelines will vary.[21]

For high-risk nodules (> 10% risk of malignancy) greater than 8 mm diameter (or 300 mm³ volume) a fludeoxyglucose positron emission tomography (FDG-PET) scan can help assess risk of malignancy. High-risk nodules identified on PET should be considered for image-guided or excision biopsy depending on patient fitness and preference. Lower-risk nodules can be followed up with interval LDCT (see page 10). Sub-solid nodules will require longer follow-up than solid nodules as they may represent premalignant adenocarcinoma in situ or minimally invasive adenocarcinoma.

Key points – prevention and screening

- Tobacco smoke exposure accounts for 90% of all lung cancers. Smoking prevention and cessation represents the major target for prevention of non-small-cell lung cancer (NSCLC).
- The National Lung Screening Trial showed that low-dose CT screening of high-risk individuals reduced the risk of lung cancer-related mortality by 20%.
- The management of solitary pulmonary nodules is dependent on their risk stratification, evidence of growth on interval imaging (ideally using volumetric measurement) and patient comorbidities and choices.

References

1. Dela Cruz CS, Tanoue LT, Matthay RA. Lung cancer: epidemiology, etiology, and prevention. *Clin Chest Med* 2011;32:605–44.

2. Ferlay J, Soerjomataram I, Ervik M et al. GLOBOCAN 2012 v1.0. Cancer incidence and mortality worldwide: IARC CancerBase No. 11 (Internet). Lyon, France: International Agency for Research on Cancer, 2013. http://globocan. iarc.fr, last accessed 01 August 2016.

3. Malvezzi M, Bertuccio P, Rosso T et al. European cancer mortality predictions for the year 2015: does lung cancer have the highest death rate in EU women? *Ann Oncol* 2015;26:779–86.

4. Surgeon General's Advisory Committee on Smoking and Health. *Smoking and Health. Report of the Advisory Committee to the Surgeon General of the Public Health Service.* Washington, DC: US Department of Health, Education and Welfare, 1964.

5. Spyratos D, Zaragoulidis P, Porpodis K et al. Occupational exposure and lung cancer. *J Thorac Dis* 2013;5:S440–5.

6. Bailey-Wilson JE, Amos CI, Pinney SM et al. A major lung cancer susceptibility locus maps to chromosome 6q23–25. *Am J Hum Genet* 2004;75:460–74.

7. Raviv S, Hawkins KA, DeCamp Jr MM, Kalhan R. Lung cancer in chronic obstructive pulmonary disease. Enhancing surgical options and outcomes. *Am J Respir Crit Care Med* 2011;183:1138–46.

8. Samet JM. Does idiopathic pulmonary fibrosis increase lung cancer risk? *Am J Respir Crit Care Med* 2000;161:1–2. [Editorial]

9. Lee JY, Jeon I, Lee JM et al. Diabetes mellitus as an independent risk factor for lung cancer: a meta-analysis of observational studies. *Eur J Cancer* 2013;49: 2411–23.

10. Ng AK, Kenney LB, Gilbert ES, Travis LB. Secondary malignancies across the age spectrum. *Semin Radiat Oncol* 2010;20:67–78.

11. Zablotska LB, Neugut AI. Lung carcinoma after radiation therapy in women treated with lumpectomy or mastectomy for primary breast carcinoma. *Cancer* 2003;97: 1404–11.

12. Engels EA, Brock MV, Chen J et al. Elevated incidence of lung cancer among HIV-infected individuals. *J Clin Oncol* 2006;24:1383–8.

13. Key TJ. Fruit and vegetables and cancer risk. *Br J Cancer* 2011;104:6–11.

14. Omenn GS, Goodman GE, Thornquist MD et al. Risk factors for lung cancer and for intervention effects in CARET, the Beta-Carotene and Retinol Efficacy Trial. *J Natl Cancer Inst* 1996;88:1550–9.

15. Bjelakovic G, Gluud LL, Nikolova D et al. Vitamin D supplementation for prevention of cancer in adults. *Cochrane Database Syst Rev* 2014;(6):CD007469.

16. Oken MM, Hocking WG, Kvale PA et al. Screening by chest radiograph and lung cancer mortality. *JAMA* 2011;306: 1865–73.

17. National Lung Screening Trial Research Team; Aberle DR, Adams AM, Berg CD et al. Reduced lung-cancer mortality with low-dose computed tomographic screening. *N Engl J Med* 2011;365:395–409.

18. Horaweg N, Scholten ET, de Jong PA et al. Detection of lung cancer through low-dose CT screening (NELSON): a prespecified analysis of screening test performance and interval cancers. *Lancet Oncol* 2014;15:1342–50.

19. Field JK, Duffy SW, Baldwin DR et al. UK Lung Cancer RCT Pilot Screening Trial: baseline findings from the screening arm provide evidence for the potential implementation of lung cancer screening. *Thorax* 2016;71:161–70.

20. Kauczor H-U, Bonomo L, Gaga M et al. ESR/ERS white paper on lung cancer screening. *Eur Respir J* 2015;46:28–39.

21. Callister MEJ, Baldwin DR, Akram AR et al. British Thoracic Society guidelines for the investigation and management of pulmonary nodules. *Thorax* 2015;70(Suppl 2):ii1–ii54.

The most common symptoms of advanced intrathoracic disease are cough, hemoptysis, dyspnea, chest pain, bronchial obstruction and dysphagia. These symptoms usually trigger a chest X-ray (CXR). Some lung cancers are identified by an abnormality found on imaging that is carried out for reasons other than chest symptoms (e.g. for employment reasons or before elective surgery). Initial evaluation of a patient after imaging should involve tissue biopsy by bronchoscopy, endobronchial ultrasound, or guided ultrasonography or CT. This information, together with radiological staging and a multidisciplinary meeting discussion usually results in a treatment plan. This plan must then be considered in terms of the patient's comorbidities (cardiac and respiratory function) and individual wishes. Every patient with suspected lung cancer should undergo a thorough history and physical examination, which, together with laboratory testing can assess comorbid conditions and the likelihood of metastases.

CT, and in some cases positron emission tomography (PET), provides a non-invasive assessment of tumor size (T), mediastinal node enlargement (N) and potential metastases (M) (see Staging, Chapter 3).

Small biopsies and cytology specimens

About 70% of patients present with advanced stage lung cancer. Diagnosis is usually made from small biopsy and cytology specimens. Historically, pathologists only needed to distinguish between small-cell lung cancer (SCLC) and non-small-cell lung cancer (NSCLC), but in recent years therapeutic and genetic advances have driven the need for larger quantities of tissue for histological subclassification, immunohistochemistry and molecular and immune pathology.[1]

The 2015 World Health Organization Classification of Tumors of the Lung, Pleura, Thymus and Heart includes a new classification for small biopsies and cytology similar to that proposed in the 2011 Association for the Study of Lung Cancer/American Thoracic Society/ European Respiratory Society classification.[2]

Well-differentiated tumors with adenocarcinoma morphology (acinar, papillary, lepidic, micropapillary) or squamous cell carcinoma (unequivocal keratinization and well-formed classical bridges) on routine light microscopy can be diagnosed as adenocarcinoma or squamous cell carcinoma, respectively, without immunohistochemistry.

Poorly differentiated tumors should undergo limited immuno-histochemistry. A single adenocarcinoma marker (e.g. thyroid transcription factor 1 [TTF1] or Napsin-A) or squamous cell carcinoma marker (e.g. p40, cytokeratin 5/6 or p63) can be used to classify most tumors.

Carcinomas lacking clear differentiation by morphology and immunohistochemistry are classified as 'NSCLC, not otherwise specified (NOS)'. NOS carcinomas that stain with adenocarcinoma markers are classified as 'NSCLC, favor adenocarcinoma'; tumors that stain with squamous markers are classified as 'NSCLC, favor squamous cell carcinoma'. In this way, a diagnosis of NSCLC–NOS can be avoided in up to 90% of cases.

Molecular testing for tumor gene (somatic) mutations

The discovery of specific gene mutations in NSCLC (Table 2.1) has led to the development of targeted therapies. In particular, the presence of epidermal growth factor receptor (*EGFR*) gene mutations, found primarily in adenocarcinomas, is predictive of responsiveness to EGFR tyrosine kinase inhibitors.[3] Furthermore, adenocarcinomas with *ALK-MET* rearrangements are responsive to crizotinib,[4] and patients with adenocarcinoma or NSCLC–NOS are more responsive to pemetrexed than are those with squamous cell carcinoma.[5] In the initial randomized phase 2 study of bevacizumab and chemotherapy in advanced NSCLC, bevacizumab was associated with life-threatening hemorrhage in patients with squamous cell carcinoma;[6] therefore, it is contraindicated in patients with this NSCLC histology.

TABLE 2.1

Frequency of gene mutations in NSCLC

Gene	Alteration	Frequency in NSCLC
EGFR	Mutation	10–35%
KRAS	Mutation	15–25%
FGFR1	Amplification	20%
PTEN	Mutation	4–8%
DDR2	Mutation	~4%
ALK	Rearrangement	3–7%
MET	Amplification	2–4%
HER2	Mutation	2–4%
BRAF	Mutation	1–3%
PIK3CA	Mutation	1–3%
AKT1	Mutation	1%
MEK1	Mutation	1%
NRAS	Mutation	1%
RET	Rearrangement	1%
ROS1	Rearrangement	1%

Source: Lovly C, Horn L, Pao W. 2016. Molecular Profiling of Lung Cancer. *My Cancer Genome* www.mycancergenome.org/content/disease/lung-cancer, last accessed 08 August 2016.

Key points – diagnosis and pathological classification

- The 2015 World Health Organization Classification of Lung Tumors recommends the use of immunohistochemistry for the classification of non-small-cell lung cancer (NSCLC).
- Classification of NSCLC further into specific pathological subtypes (e.g. adenocarcinoma versus squamous cell carcinoma) will determine eligibility for certain types of molecular testing and aid therapeutic decisions based on the specific histological and genetic characteristics of the tumor.
- An epidermal growth factor receptor (*EGFR*) mutation is a validated predictive marker for response to EGFR tyrosine kinase inhibitor treatments.

References

1. Travis WD, Brambilla E, Noguchi M et al. International Association for the Study of Lung Cancer/American Thoracic Society/European Respiratory Society International Multidisciplinary Classification of Lung Adenocarcinoma. *J Thoracic Oncol* 2011;6:244–85.

2. Travis WD, Brambilla E, Nicholson Ag et al. The 2015 World Health Organization classification of lung tumors: impact of genetic, clinical and radiologic advances since the 2004 classification. *J Thoracic Oncol* 2015;10:1243–60.

3. Bethune G, Bethune D, Ridgway N, Xu Z. Epidermal growth factor receptor (EGFR) in lung cancer: an overview and update. *J Thorac Dis* 2010;2:48–51.

4. Awad MM, Shaw AT. ALK inhibitors in non-small cell lung cancer: crizotinib and beyond. *Clin Adv Hematol Oncol* 2014;12:429–39.

5. Scagliotti G, Hanna N, Fossella F et al. The differential efficacy of pemetrexed according to NSCLC histology: a review of two Phase III studies. *Oncologist* 2009;14:253–63.

6. Johnson DH, Fehrenbacher L, Novotny WF et al. Randomized phase II trial comparing bevacizumab plus carboplatin and paclitaxel with carboplatin and paclitaxel alone in previously untreated locally advanced or metastatic non-small-cell lung cancer. *J Clin Oncol* 2004;22:2184–91.

Ilaria Onorati MD *and Olaf Mercier* MD PhD, *Department of*
Thoracic and Vascular Surgery and Heart–Lung Transplantation,
Marie Lannelongue Hospital, Thoracic Oncology Institute,
Paris-Saclay University, Le Plessis Robinson, France

TNM classification (IASLC, eighth edition)

As stage is one of the most important prognostic factors at diagnosis and is essential when making treatment decisions, it is important that it is as accurate as possible. At present, the extent of non-small-cell lung cancer (NSCLC) disease is staged according to the 2009 tumor–node–metastasis (TNM) classification (seventh edition).[1] The International Association for the Study of Lung Cancer (IASLC) has proposed several changes to be implemented in the forthcoming eighth edition, which reflect global experience in the management of NSCLC.[2]

Tumor size (T) is the primary descriptive and most significant prognostic factor for operable lung cancer. Table 3.1 shows the proposed changes to the current T classification. Subclassification of early-stage NSCLC according to the size of the tumor will allow trials to compare the survival benefit of sublobar resections (i.e. wedge resection or segmentectomy) and lobectomy (see pages 24–6). Surgical advances have enabled 'distance from the carina' to be removed from the new TNM classification.[3] However, the poor prognosis associated with pleural invasion has been confirmed, and therefore it remains a contraindication to surgery.

Nodal status (N). A fundamental prerequisite in selecting patients for surgical treatment is reliable nodal staging (Table 3.2). The current N classification of nodal staging adequately predicts prognosis, so no change to the N descriptors has been recommended in the eighth edition.[2] Division of the N1 stage into N1a (N1 at a single station) and N1b (N1 at multiple stations), and division of the N2 stage into

TABLE 3.1

Proposed 'T' classification changes for the new tumor–nodes–metastasis (TNM) staging system for NSCLC

	Primary tumor	Proposed changes
TX	Primary tumor cannot be assessed, or tumor is proven by presence of malignant cells in sputum or bronchial washing but not visualized by imaging or bronchoscopy	
Tis	Carcinoma in situ	
T1	< 3 cm in greatest dimension, surrounded by lung or visceral pleura, without bronchoscopic evidence of invasion more proximal than lobar bronchus	
T1a	≤ 2 cm	≤ 1 cm
T1b	> 2 cm but ≤ 3 cm	> 1 cm but ≤ 2 cm
		T1c > 2 cm but ≤ 3 cm
T2	> 3 cm but ≤ 7 cm, or tumor with any of: • main bronchus involvement > 2 cm distal to the carina • invasion of visceral pleura • tumor with partial atelectasis/ pneumonitis	Involvement of main bronchus regardless of distance from the carina Tumor with partial and total atelectasis/ pneumonitis
T2a	> 3 cm but ≤ 5 cm	> 3 cm but ≤ 4 cm
T2b	> 5 cm but ≤ 7 cm	> 4 cm to ≤ 5 cm
T3	> 7 cm	> 5 cm
T4	Tumor of any size that invades any of: mediastinum, heart great vessels, trachea, recurrent laryngeal nerve, carina, vertebral body or esophagus or separate nodule(s) in a different ipsilateral lobe	> 7 cm Diaphragmatic involvement

TABLE 3.2

'N' classification in the tumor–nodes–metastasis (TNM) staging system for NSCLC

NX Regional lymph nodes cannot be assessed

N0 No regional node metastasis

N1 Metastasis in ipsilateral peribronchial and/or ipsilateral hilar lymph nodes and intrapulmonary nodes, including involvement by direct extension

N2 Metastasis in ipsilateral mediastinal and/or subcarinal lymph node(s)

N3 Metastasis in contralateral mediastinal, contralateral hilar, ipsilateral or contralateral scalene or supraclavicular lymph nodes

The latest international guidelines for the treatment of N2 disease indicate that further nodal subclassification may be useful when selecting patients with N2 disease for multimodal treatment, including surgery (see Table 3.5, page 28).[4,5]

N2a1 (N2 at a single station without N1 involvement; 'skip' metastasis), N2a2 (N2 at a single station with N1 involvement) and N2b (N2 at multiple stations) is descriptive only, as the survival curves for N1b and N2a2 overlap. Although N2a1 was associated with a better prognosis than N1b, the difference was not significant.

Metastasis (M). When patients were assessed according to the number of metastases, there were no significant differences in prognosis in patients with M1a staging (metastases within the chest cavity); however, patients with M1b tumors (distant metastases outside the chest cavity) with a single metastasis in a single organ had a significantly better prognosis than those with multiple metastases in one or several organs. This will now be the definition of M1b and will serve as a first step in providing rational selection criteria for surgical treatment of oligometastatic disease in clinical trials.[4] There will also be a new M1c classification (Table 3.3) – multiple metastases in a single organ or in multiple organs.

TABLE 3.3

Proposed 'M' classification changes for the new tumor–nodes–metastasis (TNM) staging system for NSCLC

TNM 2009	M (metastatic disease)	Proposed changes
MX	Distant metastasis cannot be assessed	
M0	No distant metastasis	
M1a	Chest cavity metastasis	
M1b	Distant metastases outside the chest cavity	M1b Single distant metastasis outside the chest cavity M1c Multiple metastases in a single organ or in multiple organs

Surgical resection of early-stage NSCLC

Surgery is the gold standard treatment for early-stage (I and II) lung cancer (Table 3.4).

Surgical procedures[5] continue to evolve along a 'less is more' trajectory, with an increasing trend toward minimally invasive techniques (video-assisted thoracoscopic surgery [VATS] or robotics) and the removal of as little lung parenchyma as possible (lobectomy > segmentectomy > wedge resection; Figure 3.1).

Minimally invasive surgery versus open surgery. Minimally invasive procedures for early-stage NSCLC have become standard and an alternative to open surgery in centers with the appropriate experience. In a recent meta-analysis, patients who underwent VATS lobectomy had a significantly lower incidence of postoperative prolonged air leak, pneumonia, atrial arrhythmias and renal failure, and a shorter duration of hospital stay than those who had a thoracotomy.[6] Furthermore, patients who underwent VATS had significantly higher adherence to adjuvant chemotherapy (earlier onset and higher completion rate) than those who underwent thoracotomy.[7] However,

TABLE 3.4

Antatomic staging for NSCLC based on tumor–nodes–metastasis (TNM) classifications*

Stage	T	N	M
Ia	T1a, T1b, T1c	N0	M0
Ib	T2a	N0	M0
IIa	T1a, T1b, T2a	N1	M0
	T2b	N0	M0
IIb	T2b	N1	M0
	T3	N0	M0
IIIa	T1, T2	N2	M0
	T3	N1	M0
	T4	N0, N1	M0
IIIb	T1, T2, T3	N3	M0
	T4	N2, N3	M0
IV	T Any	N Any	M1a, M1b, M1c

*See Tables 3.1, 3.2 and 3.3.

there was no difference in oncologic results or lung function recovery during the late postoperative period.[8]

Interest in robotic lung surgery for NSCLC is rising even though it has not demonstrated superiority over VATS with respect to the length of hospital stay.[9] Further studies may help to determine the role of robotic surgery in NSCLC in the future.

Wedge resection versus segmentectomy versus lobectomy. The type of resection (see Figure 3.1) selected for the treatment of T1aN0M0 tumors depends on the patient's age, cardiopulmonary reserve, tumor size and histology.

A review of 45 prospective and retrospective studies conducted over the last 25 years showed that segmentectomies are superior to wedge resections in terms of local recurrences and cancer-related mortality

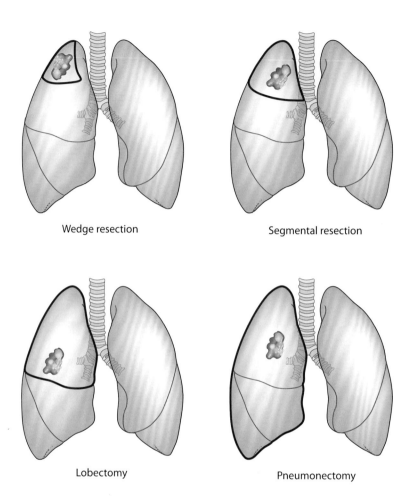

Wedge resection

Segmental resection

Lobectomy

Pneumonectomy

Figure 3.1 The surgical options for NSCLC.

rates.[10] Whether the long-term results of lung-sparing segmentectomies and lobectomies are equivalent has yet to be determined. Lobectomies had better results than segmentectomies for tumors greater than 2 cm in diameter (T2bN0M0) in terms of disease-free and overall 5-year survival.[10,11] In general, recent studies have failed to show any difference in survival outcomes between lobectomies, segmentectomies and wedge resections for small tumors less than 2 cm,[12] although patients with invasive adenocarcinoma less than 2 cm may have improved survival outcomes after segmentectomy.[13] The results of

25

randomized clinical trials are awaited to determine if segmentectomies may be the preferred surgical treatment for the new classifications of T1a and T1b N0M0 tumors. Segmentectomies may also be considered in high-risk patients, or in the case of pure bronchoalveolar carcinomas for lung-sparing purposes.

Regardless of their extent, lung resections must comply with the principles of oncologic surgery in terms of disease-free margins and adequate systematic lymphadenectomy.

Ground glass opacity (GGO) is a pulmonary shadow visualized using high-resolution computed tomography (HRCT), comprised of hazy increased attenuation with preservation of the bronchial and vascular margins. Adenocarcinoma is the most common cause of GGO, therefore careful evaluation for pulmonary malignancy must be considered when GGO is identified.[14]

Patients with multiple tumors and a prominent ground glass component on imaging or lepidic component on microscopy are being seen with increasing frequency. These tumors are associated with good survival after resection and have a lower propensity for nodal and extrathoracic spread than other types of NSCLC; however, they frequently relapse. Sublobar resection with the goal of sparing lung parenchyma is the gold standard for treatment of small GGO. The main difficulty is localizing the tumor within the lung during minimally invasive surgery. Different means of tracking the GGO and guiding the resection have been studied, including ink injection, coil insertion, and indocianide green injection.[15-17]

Diffuse pneumonic-type involvement has a worse prognosis; it can lead to severe hypoxemia and end-stage respiratory distress. In this setting, a lobectomy is preferable to sublobar resection. In cases of bilateral pneumonic-type involvement with deep hypoxemia, lung transplantation has been studied in specifically selected patients with a high-risk of recurrence, with limited results.[18]

For multifocal ground glass/lepidic tumors, the IASLC proposes that T staging should be defined by the largest T lesion, with either the number of tumors or 'm' in parentheses to denote the multifocal nature of the condition, and a single N and M category defining all the lesions collectively; for example, T1a(3)N0M0 or T1a(m)N0M0. For diffuse pneumonic-type lung cancer, T staging is designated by the tumor size if it is within one lobe, or as T4 if it involves an ipsilateral different lobe, or M1a if it is contralateral. A single N and M category is used for all pulmonary areas of involvement.[2]

Surgical resection of locally advanced NSCLC

Most lung cancers are detected at an advanced stage and are treated with chemotherapy and radiotherapy. Surgical resection has proved valuable in a subset of patients with advanced NSCLC without nodal involvement or distant metastasis, resulting in long-term survival with a lower risk of postoperative mortality. Surgery also has a relevant role in the treatment of locally advanced tumors invading neighboring structures.

Patients with locally advanced NSCLC (T3 and T4 tumors) should be treated with multimodality therapy. Advances in perioperative management and postoperative care along with careful patient selection, are likely to make the operative mortality and morbidity less prohibitive. The prognosis after operations for T4 tumors mainly depends on the N stage and completeness of the resection. Patients with N0 or minimal N1 disease and complete resection do significantly better after radical resection than patients with N2 disease.[19] The European and US guidelines for treatment of N2 disease are shown in Table 3.5.

Improvement of surgical techniques and anesthesiology has led to extended resection procedures such as carinal resections, chest wall resection with reconstruction, Pancoast tumor resections, vascular resections and reconstruction and spine resection, with low postoperative mortality and long-term survival of up to 50% at 5 years. In the present staging system, T4N0–1M0 lesions are categorized as stage IIIA disease (see Table 3.4), and T4 tumors without mediastinal nodal metastasis are now considered to be potentially curable if complete resection is possible.[2]

For patients with resectable stage III NSCLC, the optimal treatment strategy remains unclear. Further clinical trials are needed to clarify the timing of surgery as part of multimodal treatment for resectable stage IIIA NSCLC.[20,21]

TABLE 3.5

European and US guidelines for N2 disease treatment

Europe	USA
Consider radical radiotherapy or chemoradiotherapy in patients with T1–4N2 (bulky or fixed) M0 disease	In patients with discrete N2 involvement by NSCLC identified preoperatively (IIIA), either definitive chemoradiation therapy or induction therapy followed by surgery is recommended over either surgery or radiation alone
Consider surgery as part of multimodal management of patients with T1–3N2 (non-fixed, non-bulky, single zone) M0 disease	In patients with NSCLC who have incidental (occult) N2 disease (IIIA) found at surgical resection despite thorough preoperative staging and in whom complete resection of the lymph nodes and primary tumor is technically possible, completion of the planned lung resection and mediastinal lymphadenectomy is suggested
Consider further randomized trials of surgery added to multimodal management of patients with multizone N2 disease to establish if any subgroups of patients might benefit more from the addition of surgery	

Key points – staging and surgery

- Better subclassification of early-stage NSCLC according to the size of the tumor will allow trials to compare wedge resection and segmentectomy.
- New M1c staging for multiple metastases in one or several organs and the use of the term M1b for oligometastatic disease has the potential to provide rational selection criteria for clinical treatment trials.
- Ground glass opacity (GGO) visualized on high-resolution computed tomography should trigger careful evaluation for pulmonary malignancy.
- Some locally advanced lung cancers benefit from multimodality therapy, which can include surgery.

References

1. Tanoue LT, Detterbeck FC. New TNM classification for non-small-cell lung cancer. *Expert Rev Anticancer Ther* 2009;9:413–23.

2. Goldstraw P, Chansky K, Crowley J et al. The IASLC Lung Cancer Staging Project: proposals for revision of the TNM stage groupings in the forthcoming (eighth) edition of the TNM Classification for Lung Cancer. *J Thorac Oncol* 2016; 11:39–51.

3. Weder W, Inci I. Carinal resection and sleeve pneumonectomy. *Thorac Surg Clin* 2014;24:77–83.

4. Lim E, Baldwin D, Beckles M et al. Guidelines on the radical management of patients with lung cancer. *Thorax* 2010;65 Suppl 3:iii1–27.

5. Howington JA, Blum MG, Chang AC et al. Treatment of stage I and II non-small cell lung cancer: diagnosis and management of lung cancer, 3rd ed: American College of Chest Physicians evidence-based clinical practice guidelines. *Chest* 2013;143:e278S–313S.

6. Cao C, Manganas C, Ang SC et al. Video-assisted thoracic surgery versus open thoracotomy for non-small cell lung cancer: a meta-analysis of propensity score-matched patients. *Interact Cardiovasc Thorac Surg* 2013;16:244–9.

7. Teh E, Abah U, Church D et al. What is the extent of the advantage of video-assisted thoracoscopic surgical resection over thoracotomy in terms of delivery of adjuvant chemotherapy following non-small-cell lung cancer resection? *Interact Cardiovasc Thorac Surg* 2014;19:656–60.

8. Park TY, Park YS. Long-term respiratory function recovery in patients with stage I lung cancer receiving video-assisted thoracic surgery versus thoracotomy. *J Thorac Dis* 2016;8:161–8.

9. Yang HX, Woo KM, Sima CS et al. Long-term survival based on the surgical approach to lobectomy for clinical stage I nonsmall cell lung cancer: comparison of robotic, video-assisted thoracic surgery, and thoracotomy lobectomy. *Ann Surg* 2016;Mar 22. [ePub ahead of print]

10. Reveliotis K, Kalavrouziotis G, Skevis K et al. Wedge resection and segmentectomy in patients with stage I non-small cell lung carcinoma. *Oncol Rev* 2014;8:234–41.

11. Ginsberg RJ, Rubinstein LV. Randomized trial of lobectomy versus limited resection for T1 N0 non-small cell lung cancer. Lung Cancer Study Group. *Ann Thorac Surg* 1995;60:615–22.

12. Razi SS, John MM, Sainathan S, Stavropoulos C. Sublobar resection is equivalent to lobectomy for T1a non-small cell lung cancer in the elderly: a Surveillance, Epidemiology, and End Results database analysis. *J Surg Res* 2016;200:683–9.

13. Zhang Y, Sun Y, Chen H. A propensity score matching analysis of survival following segmentectomy or wedge resection in early-stage lung invasive adenocarcinoma or squamous cell carcinoma. *Oncotarget* 2016;7:13880–5.

14. Pedersen JH, Saghir Z, Wille MM et al. Ground-glass opacity lung nodules in the era of lung cancer CT screening: radiology, pathology, and clinical management. *Oncology (Williston Park)* 2016;30:266–74.

15. Keating JJ, Kennedy GT, Singhal S. Identification of a subcentimeter pulmonary adenocarcinoma using intraoperative near-infrared imaging during video-assisted thoracoscopic surgery. *J Thorac Cardiovasc Surg* 2015;149:e51–3.

16. Kim HK, Quan YH, Choi BH et al. Intraoperative pulmonary neoplasm identification using near-infrared fluorescence imaging. *Eur J Cardiothorac Surg* 2015;49:1497–502.

17. Sato M, Yamada T, Menju T et al. Virtual-assisted lung mapping: outcome of 100 consecutive cases in a single institute. *Eur J Cardiothorac Surg* 2015;47:e131–9.

18. de Perrot M, Chernenko S, Waddell TK et al. Role of lung transplantation in the treatment of bronchogenic carcinomas for patients with end-stage pulmonary disease. *J Clin Oncol* 2004;22:4351–6.

19. Yildizeli B, Dartevelle PG, Fadel E et al. Results of primary surgery with T4 non-small cell lung cancer during a 25-year period in a single center: the benefit is worth the risk. *Ann Thorac Surg* 2008;86:1065–75.

20. Yokoi K, Taniguchi T, Usami N et al. Surgical management of locally advanced lung cancer. *Gen Thorac Cardiovasc Surg* 2014;62:522–30.

21. Antoni D, Mornex F. Chemoradiotherapy of locally advanced nonsmall cell lung cancer: state of the art and perspectives. *Curr Opin Oncol* 2016;28:104–9.

4 Radiotherapy

Paul Kabuubi MBChB MRCP FRCR *and Merina Ahmed* BSc MBBS MRCP
FRCR MD(Res), *The Royal Marsden NHS Foundation Trust, London, UK*

Radiotherapy has a role in the management of most patients with non-small-cell lung cancer (NSCLC). While it can be used as sole treatment, it is often integrated in a multimodal strategy with surgery and chemotherapy.[1] Overall, treatment options vary according to the stage of the tumor (see Chapter 3) but also depend on the individual patient's lung function, volume of disease and performance status.

Patient selection

To be eligible for radical radiotherapy, patients must have adequate lung function (forced expiratory volume in 1 second [FEV_1] $\geq$ 1 liter or $\geq$ 40% predicted; transfer factor $\geq$ 40%), good performance status (Eastern Cooperative Oncology Group [ECOG] score 0–1) and disease that can be encompassed in a radiotherapy treatment volume without undue risk of damaging normal tissue. Patients with interstitial lung disease are rarely suitable. Patients with poor lung function may still be eligible provided they have been adequately counseled about the long-term risks of breathlessness. Unsuitable candidates for radical radiotherapy should be offered other palliative options.

Radical radiotherapy delivery

All patients eligible for radiotherapy should first undergo a planning CT scan in the treatment position. The target volume is defined using information acquired from diagnostic contrast-enhanced CT and fludeoxyglucose–positron emission tomography (FDG-PET) scans. Mediastinoscopy is required to aid nodal definition if the CT and PET findings are inconclusive. As the tumor can move, respiratory motion management is mandatory when planning and treating the patient. The planned target volume then accounts for any tumor excursion.

Modern techniques used to deliver radical radiotherapy include three-dimensional (3D) conformal radiotherapy, intensity-modulated

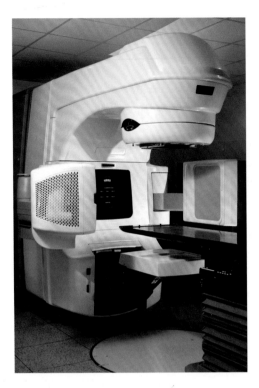

Figure 4.1 Linear accelerator (Linac). Standard radiotherapy machine used for the majority of lung radiotherapy treatments.

radiotherapy (IMRT) and volumetric arc therapy (VMAT) (Figure 4.1).

Conventionally, fractionated radiotherapy is administered, usually with a daily dose of approximately 2 Gy. Hyperfractionation is radiotherapy delivered at less than 2 Gy per fraction but more than once a day so that the treatment time remains the same but total dose is increased. Hypofractionated radiotherapy refers to dose fractions greater than 2 Gy and allows acceleration of treatment. Hypo- or hyperfractionated treatment have the potential for increased late toxicity.

The principal schedules are:
- conventional fractionation: 64–66 Gy in 32–33 daily fractions over 6.5 weeks
- accelerated hypofractionation: 55 Gy in 20 fractions over 4 weeks
- continuous hyperfractionated accelerated radiotherapy (CHART): 54 Gy in 36 fractions over 12 consecutive days.

Conventional fractionation and accelerated hypofractionation are thought to be equivalent, but hypofractionation involves fewer visits, is more convenient for patients and requires fewer resources.

Observational data suggest that radiotherapy is inferior to contemporary surgical series, which have reported 5-year survival of 80% for stage Ia and 60% for stage Ib.[2] Reports from cohorts who received conventionally fractionated radiotherapy indicate dismal 5-year survivals of 32% for stage I and 21% for stage II patients. In one series, this translated into a 7-month median survival advantage (21 vs 14 months) over no treatment in stage I patients and a 5-month survival advantage (14 vs 9 months) in stage II patients.[3]

CHART shortens the overall treatment time but delivers three treatment fractions per day. Compared with conventional fractionation at a dose of 60 Gy in 30 fractions, it has demonstrated superior local control (23% vs 16%) and 5-year overall survival (30% vs 21%).[4] Its implementation has been hampered by resource considerations and lack of evidence of superiority to contemporary radiation doses which are typically greater than 64 Gy.

Side effects are predominantly lung related (Table 4.1). Lung toxicity manifests as pneumonitis or inflammation in the lung (less than 6 months), usually presenting as a cough or dyspnea. Myelitis is rare.

Stereotactic body radiotherapy (SBRT) or stereotactic ablative radiotherapy is the delivery of an extremely high dose of radiotherapy to a small target using hypofractionation. The fraction sizes are typically greater than 8 Gy per fraction. It is used for the treatment of stage I disease, and more recently for the treatment of oligometastatic disease. Methods of delivery are shown in Table 4.2. Image-guided radiotherapy (IGRT) refers to the use of imaging to reduce the uncertainty of tumor position during treatment.

It has been estimated that a dose greater than 84 Gy is needed to provide 50% tumor control at 3 years.[5] A meta-analysis in stage I patients has confirmed equivalent survival to surgery at 2 years.[6] Local failures occur in less than 10% of patients but these failure rates can increase as tumor volume increases, with T2 disease or as the dose falls.

TABLE 4.1

Short- and long-term side effects of radiotherapy for NSCLC

	Radical conventional RT	SBRT	Palliative RT
Acute side effects	Fatigue	Fatigue	Fatigue
	Dyspnea	Dyspnea	Dyspnea
	Esophagitis	Esophagitis	Esophagitis
	Skin reaction	Skin reaction	Skin reaction
	Cough	Cough	
		Chest wall pain	
Late side effects	Lung fibrosis	Lung fibrosis	Lung fibrosis
	Reduction in breathing capacity	Reduction in breathing capacity	Risk of nerve damage (< 1%)
	Risk of cardiac damage	Risk of cardiac damage	
	Risk of nerve damage (< 1%)	Risk of nerve damage (< 1%)	
	Risk of swallowing problems (very low)	Skin necrosis (easily avoided with careful planning)	
		Rib fracture (10–40%) or chest wall pain	
		Tracheal/bronchial fistula*	
		Pulmonary hemorrhage*	

*For central tumors only. RT, radiotherapy; SBRT, stereotactic body radiotherapy.

The indications for SBRT over other radiotherapy techniques are shown in Table 4.3 and Figure 4.2. Patients can be treated without histological confirmation if there is consensus at multidisciplinary meetings that the radiologically evident tumor shows incremental growth and abnormal PET avidity.

TABLE 4.2

Modern modes of radiotherapy delivery

| | Technological development in NSCLC → | | | | | |
	3D conformal RT	Intensity-modulated RT	Tomotherapy	Volumetric arc therapy	Stereotactic RT	Image-guided RT
Description	Irregularly shaped co-planar fields of uniform intensity	Irregularly shaped non-planar fields of varying intensity	Helical IMRT integrated with CT scanner	IMRT delivered with a rotating gantry on a Linac	Very high dose to small target	RT that adapts to changes in tumor position, size and shape
Conformality*	+	++	++	++	++++	+++
Number of fields	3–4 fixed	5–7	1 helix	1–2 arcs	–	As per method of delivery
Size of low-dose bath†	+	+++	++++	++++	+	–
Duration of treatment	5–10 mins/fraction	10–15 mins/fraction	5 mins/fraction	5 mins/fraction	15–90 mins/fraction	10–20 mins/fraction

*Conformality is the similarity between the target and the three-dimensional shape of the high-dose distribution.
†The splash of low dose outside the target has a theoretical link to the risk of secondary malignancy.
CT, computed tomography; IMRT, intensity-modulated radiotherapy; Linac, linear accelerator (see Figure 4.1); RT, radiotherapy.

TABLE 4.3

Eligibility for stereotactic body radiotherapy

- Stage T1a, T1b, T2a (some centers treat T2b disease, but local control rates diminish as volume increases)
- Tumor is located outside of the 'no-fly zone' (Figure 4.2)*
- Medically inoperable or patient declines surgery, PS 0–2
- No interstitial lung disease

*Some centers treat central tumors within this no fly zone with a more modest hypofractionated regimen. In experienced hands, side effects are minimal as the dose to surrounding organs is low.
PS, performance status.

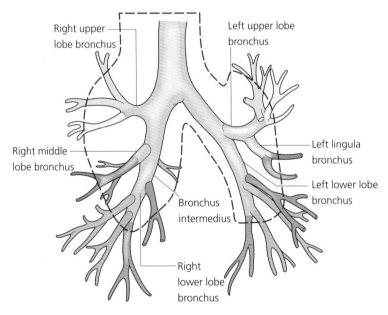

Figure 4.2 'No fly zone' as published by Radiation Therapy and Oncology Group (RTOG) guidelines.

Radical radiotherapy with chemotherapy. The best outcomes are seen when conventional radical radiotherapy is used concurrently with chemotherapy; in a meta-analysis of 1764 patients with stage IIIA and IIIB disease, the absolute benefit of concurrent chemoradiation over radical radiotherapy alone was 4% and 2.2% at 2 years and 5 years, respectively, with increased risk of grade 3/4 esophagitis.[7]

Sequential chemoradiation (chemotherapy before radiotherapy), or occasionally radiotherapy alone, is recommended for patients with a relatively large tumor volume or for patients not fit enough to receive concurrent chemoradiation. The sequential versus concurrent approach gives 5-year survival rates of 18% vs 23%, respectively.[8]

Dose intensification

The CHART regimen of hyperfractionated accelerated treatment has shown a survival benefit over standard radical radiotherapy delivery.[4]

The RTOG trial 0617 indicated that dose escalation was detrimental,[9] although the trial has been criticized for suboptimal radiotherapy quality assurance and a high number of protocol violations.

The SOCCAR trial (55 Gy in 20 fractions) demonstrated that hypofractionated accelerated radiotherapy can be given safely with concurrent chemotherapy.[10] This hypofractionated radiotherapy regimen, widely used in the UK, will form the basis of the control arm in the upcoming UK ADSCAN trial, which will assess dose intensification in sequential chemoradiation.

Postoperative radiotherapy

Postoperative radiotherapy (PORT) has a role in reducing the risk of recurrence in patients who are found to have a positive margin on histopathology, i.e. residual microscopic disease (an R1 resection), but not after R0 resections. A meta-analysis of nine randomized controlled trials over 30 years found a 7% decrease in survival (48% vs 55%, $p<0.001$) when PORT was administered.[11] This was attributed to cardiovascular and respiratory toxicity. An update in 2005 found no adverse effect in pN2 disease.[12]

The role of contemporary PORT in N2 disease is being assessed in the European LungART trial.

Palliative radiotherapy

Radiotherapy provides effective palliation of symptomatic advanced intrathoracic disease and metastases. Three randomized trials conducted by the UK's Medical Research Council (MRC) have assessed fractionation for palliation of intrathoracic symptoms.[13–15] Even when a single fraction is used, radiotherapy can produce complete resolution of symptoms in around 50% of cases.

When considering palliation of cough, chest pain and hemoptysis in those with moderate or poor performance status, 17 Gy in 2 fractions is equivalent to longer schedules (e.g. 30 Gy in 10 or 27 Gy in 6 fractions) with no difference in survival. One of the MRC trials established that 10 Gy in 1 fraction was equally effective as the 2-fraction schedule with substantially less dysphagia and no risk to the spinal cord.[13]

Patients with advanced disease who received a schedule of 39 Gy in 13 fractions showed a 2-month survival advantage over 17 Gy in 2 fractions (7 vs 9 months); however, two of the patients in the 39 Gy group and one in the 17 Gy group exhibited radiation myelopathy.[15] A dose of 36 Gy in 12 fractions is below spinal cord tolerance and therefore widely used as a safer alternative. In practice, 20 Gy in 5 fractions is frequently used in patients with performance status 2/3.

Key points – radiotherapy

- Surgery is the preferred treatment for all patients with early-stage (I–II) NSCLC, with radiotherapy reserved for those unsuitable for surgery.
- Stereotactic body radiotherapy is an alternative to surgery in peripheral stage I–II tumors less than 5 cm.
- Concurrent chemoradiotherapy is preferred to sequential chemoradiotherapy in stage IIB–IIIB disease.
- Postoperative radiotherapy is recommended when residual disease is present; it can also be discussed in patients with complete resections with pN2 disease.
- Patients with advanced disease and poor performance status should receive 10 Gy in 1 fraction for palliation of intrathoracic disease.

References

1. NSCLC Meta-analyses Collaborative Group. Adjuvant chemotherapy, with or without postoperative radiotherapy, in operable non-small-cell lung cancer: two meta-analyses of individual patient data. *Lancet* 2010;375: 1267–77.

2. Asamura H, Goya T, Koshiishi Y et al. A Japanese Lung Cancer Registry Study: prognosis of 13,010 resected lung cancers. *J Thoracic Oncol* 2008;3:46–52.

3. Wisnivesky JP, Bonomi M, Henschke C et al. Radiation therapy for the treatment of unresected stage I-II non-small cell lung cancer. *Chest* 2005;128:1461–7.

4. Saunders M, Dische S, Barrett A et al. Continuous, hyperfractionated, accelerated radiotherapy (CHART) versus conventional radiotherapy in non-small cell lung cancer: mature data from the randomised multicentre trial. *Radiother Oncol* 1999;52:137–48.

5. Martel MK, Ten Haken RK, Hazuka MB et al. Estimation of tumor control probability model parameters from 3-D dose distributions of non-small cell lung cancer patients. *Lung Cancer* 1999;24:31–7.

6. Soldà F, Lodge M, Ashley S et al. Stereotactic radiotherapy (SABR) for the treatment of primary non-small cell lung cancer; systematic review and comparison with a surgical cohort. *Radiother Oncol* 2013;109:1–7.

7. Aupérin A, Le Péchoux C, Pignon JP et al. Concomitant radio-chemotherapy based on platin compounds in patients with locally advanced non-small cell lung cancer (NSCLC): a meta-analysis of individual data from 1764 patients. *Ann Oncol* 2006;17:473–83.

8. Aupérin A, Le Péchoux C, Rolland E et al. Meta-analysis of concomitant versus sequential radiochemotherapy in locally advanced non–small-cell lung cancer. *J Clin Oncol* 2010;28:2181–90.

9. Bradley JD, Paulus R, Komaki R et al. Standard-dose versus high-dose conformal radiotherapy with concurrent and consolidation carboplatin plus paclitaxel with or without cetuximab for patients with stage IIIA or IIIB non-small-cell lung cancer (RTOG 0617): a randomised, two-by-two factorial phase 3 study. *Lancet Oncol* 2015;16:187–99.

10. Maguire J, Khan I, McMenemin R et al. SOCCAR: a randomised phase II trial comparing sequential versus concurrent chemotherapy and radical hypofractionated radiotherapy in patients with inoperable stage III non-small cell lung cancer and good performance status. *Eur J Cancer* 2014;50:2939–49.

11. PORT Meta-analysis Trialists Group. Postoperative radiotherapy in non-small-cell lung cancer: systematic review and meta-analysis of individual patient data from nine randomised controlled trials. *Lancet* 1998;352:257–63.

12. Burdett Stewart L. Postoperative radiotherapy in non-small-cell lung cancer: update of an individual patient data meta-analysis. *Lung Cancer* 2005;47:81–3.

13. Medical Research Council Lung Cancer Working Party. A Medical Research Council (MRC) randomised trial of palliative radiotherapy with two fractions or a single fraction in patients with inoperable non-small-cell lung cancer (NSCLC) and poor performance status. *Br J Cancer* 1992;65:934–41.

14. Medical Research Council Lung Cancer Working Party. Inoperable non-small-cell lung cancer (NSCLC): a Medical Research Council randomised trial of palliative radiotherapy with two fractions or ten fractions. *Br J Cancer* 1991;63:265–70.

15. Macbeth FR, Bolger JJ, Hopwood P et al.; Medical Research Council Lung Cancer Working Party. Randomized trial of palliative two-fraction versus More Intensive 13-Fraction radiotherapy for patients with inoperable non-small cell lung cancer and good performance status. *Clin Oncol* 1996;8:167–75.

Rajiv Kumar FRACP MBChB BMedSc, The Royal Marsden NHS Foundation Trust, London, UK; and Jordi Remon MD, Medical Oncology Department, Gustave Roussy, Villejuif, France

In general, non-small-cell lung cancer (NSCLC) is associated with tumor DNA damage and mutations induced by carcinogens in tobacco smoke. In the mid-1990s an antibody to one of the murine immune checkpoints was found to cure tumors in vivo.[1] The first antibody to cytotoxic T-lymphocyte-associated protein 4 (CTLA-4) was licensed 15 years later for the treatment of melanoma. This reignited the pursuit of immunotherapies in the management of cancer, including NSCLC.[2] Known as immune checkpoint inhibitors, these therapies target the programmed cell death 1 (PD-1) receptor, programmed cell death ligand-1 (PD-L1) and the CTLA-4 receptor.

Mechanism of action

PD-1 is an inhibitory cell-surface receptor that is expressed on activated T cells, B cells, natural killer cells, monocytes and dendritic cells. The effector function of T cells that express PD-1 in the tumor microenvironment can be suppressed when PD-1 is coupled to the ligand PD-L1 (B7-H1) or PD-L2 (B7-DC) on tumor cells, thus preventing an immune attack on the cancer.[3] The PD-L1 and PD-L2 ligands cross-compete for PD-1 binding; although PD-L2 has a sixfold higher binding affinity for PD-1, it has lower levels of expression, so that PD-L1 is the best ligand to target. Inhibition of the PD-1/PD-L1 immune checkpoint using monoclonal antibodies (mAbs) prevents the inhibition of the effector T-cell function, allowing T cells to maintain their tumor cell killing function (Figure 5.1).[4]

Drugs in development

Several drugs are in development (Table 5.1). The PD-1 inhibitors are immunoglobulin (Ig)G4 isotypes, while the PD-L1 inhibitors are IgG1 isotypes and are able to bind C1q and activate the complement

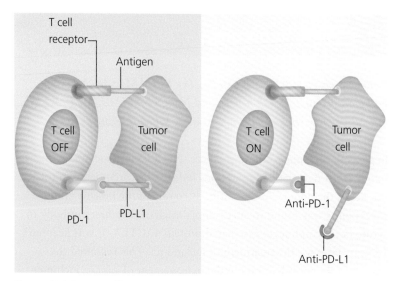

Figure 5.1 Tumor cells can present antigen to activated T cells. Upon T cell activation, programmed cell death 1 (PD-1) receptors are expressed on T cells. When coupled to the programmed cell death ligand 1 (PD-L1) receptor on the tumor cell, the normal immune response is inhibited, preventing an attack on the tumor cell. Therefore, monoclonal antibody (mAb)-mediated blockade of the PD-1/PD-L1 pathway prevents inhibition of T-cell function and enhances anti-tumor immunity.

pathway. The Fc region of naturally occurring IgG1 is able to induce antibody-dependent cell-mediated cytotoxicity (ADCC) and complement-dependent cytotoxicity (CDC), while the Fc portion of IgG4, in general, does not. However, this function is generally engineered out of Fc regions, because ADCC, when binding to the PD-1/PD-L1 axis, could potentially cause increased toxicity through killing immune cells expressing PD-1/PD-L1 and be potentially less effective. Avelumab is one of the antibodies that has retained the ADCC function.

PD-L1 expression (see Table 5.1) has been an early biomarker that has not found its true prognostic value.[5,6] The highest level of PD-L1 expression (more than 50% of tumor cells) appears to have the greatest predictive value, which is seen in about 30% of NSCLC tumors (see page 47).

TABLE 5.1

Immune checkpoint inhibitors in clinical development

Drug	Other names during development	Trade name	Class of agent	PD-L1 companion diagnostic test
PD-1 inhibitors				
Pembrolizumab	MK-3475, lambrolizumab	Keytruda	Humanized, IgG4 isotype mAb against PD-1	Test: PD-L1 IHC 22C3 Dako Membranous staining of PD-L1 on tumor cells using IHC
Nivolumab	ONO-4538, BMS-936558, MDX1106	Opdivo	Fully humanized, IgG4 isotype mAb against PD-1	Test: PD-L1 IHC 28-8 Dako Membranous staining of PD-L1 on tumor cells using IHC
PD-L1 inhibitors				
Atezolizumab	MPDL3280A	Tecentriq	Humanized, IgG1 isotype mAb against PD-L1	Test: SP142 clone – Roche in house PD-L1 expression on tumor cells and/or infiltrating lymphocytes using IHC

CONTINUED

TABLE 5.1 (CONTINUED)

Drug	Other names during development	Trade name	Class of agent	PD-L1 companion diagnostic test
Durvalumab	MEDI4736	–	Fully humanized, IgG1 isotype mAb against PD-L1	Test: SP263 clone Membranous staining of PD-L1 on tumor cells using IHC
Avelumab	MSB0010718C	–	Fully humanized, IgG1 isotype mAb against PD-L1. May induce ADCC	Not available
CTLA-4 antagonists				
Ipilimumab	MDX-010, MDX-101	Yervoy	IgG1 isotype mAb against CTLA-4	Not available
Tremelimumab	Ticilimumab, CP-675,206	–	Fully humanized, IgG2 mAb against CTLA-4	Not available

ADCC, antibody-dependent cell-mediated cytotoxicity; CTLA-4, cytotoxic T-lymphocyte associated protein 4; Ig, immunoglobulin; IHC, immunohistochemistry; mAb, monoclonal antibody; PD-1, programmed cell death protein 1; PD-L1, programmed cell death ligand-1.

Second-line monotherapy in NSCLC

Nivolumab, a fully humanized IgG4 PD-1 mAb, is licensed as second-line monotherapy for NSCLC of squamous cell histology; the approval for non-squamous histological subtypes will follow soon on the basis of the CHECKMATE-017 and CHECKMATE-057 trials.[7,8] In 272 patients with pretreated advanced squamous NSCLC, nivolumab demonstrated a significant improvement in overall response rate (ORR), progression-free survival (PFS) and overall survival (OS) compared with docetaxel, with a 1-year OS of 42% versus 24%, respectively (Table 5.2).[7] The benefits of nivolumab were independent of clinical and tumor characteristics, including PD-L1 expression.

TABLE 5.2

Seminal studies in the development of PD-1/PD-L1 inhibitors in the management of second-line NSCLC

	CHECKMATE-017[7]		
	Nivolumab	Docetaxel	
Median OS (mo)	9.2	6.0	HR=0.59, p<0.001
1-year OS	42%	24%	
ORR	20%	8%	p=0.008
Median PFS (mo)	3.5	2.8	HR=0.62, p<0.001
Median DOR (mo)	NA	8.4	
Grade 3–4 AE	7%	55%	
	CHECKMATE-057[8]		
	Nivolumab	Docetaxel	
Median OS (mo)	12.2	9.4	HR=0.73, p=0.0012
1-year OS	51%	39%	
ORR	19%	12%	p=0.02
Median PFS (mo)	2.3	4.2	HR=0.92, p=0.39
Median DOR (mo)	17.2	5.6	
Grade 3–4 AE	10%	54%	

CONTINUED

TABLE 5.2 (CONTINUED)

| | KEYNOTE-010[10] Pembrolizumab | | Docetaxel (Doc) | |
	2 mg/ kg	10 mg/ kg		
Median OS (mo)	10.4	12.7	8.5	2 mg/kg vs Doc: HR=0.71, p=0.0008
				10 mg/kg vs Doc: HR=0.61, p<0.0001
Median PFS (mo)	3.9	4.0	4.0	NS
PD-L1+ Median OS (mo)	14.9	17.3	8.2	2 mg/kg vs Doc: HR=0.54, p =0.0002
				10 mg/kg vs Doc: HR=0.50, p <0.0001
PD-L1+ Median PFS (mo)	5.0	5.2	4.1	2 mg/kg vs Doc: HR=0.59, p=0.0001
				10mg/kg vs Doc: HR=0.59, p<0.0001
ORR	18%	18%	9%	
PD-L1+ ORR	30%	29%	8%	
Grade 3–5 AE	13%	16%	35%	

	POPLAR study (Phase 2)[11] Atezolizumab	Docetaxel	
Median OS (mo)	12.6	9.7	HR=0.73, p=0.04
PD-L1+ Median OS (mo)	15.5	9.2	HR=0.59, p=0.005
Median PFS (mo)	2.7	3.0	HR=0.94, p>0.05
PD-L1+ Median PFS (mo)	2.8	3.0	HR=0.85, p>0.05
ORR	15%	15%	
PD-L1+ ORR	18%	17%	
Grade 3–4 AE	11%	39%	

AE, adverse events; DOR, duration of response; HR, hazard ratio; mo, months; ORR, overall response rate; OS, overall survival; PD-1, programmed cell death protein 1; PD-L1, programmed cell death ligand-1; PFS, progression-free survival.

In 582 patients with non-squamous NSCLC, nivolumab improved OS and ORR but not PFS (see Table 5.2). The treatment effect was consistent in all patient subgroups, especially in PD-L1-positive tumors, except for never-smokers and those with epidermal growth factor receptor (EGFR)-mutant tumors.[8]

Pembrolizumab, a highly selective, humanized IgG4 PD-1 mAb, is also licensed as second-line monotherapy for all pathological subtypes of NSCLC that express PD-L1, following the results of the KEYNOTE-001 and KEYNOTE-010 trials.[9,10] In 1034 patients with previously treated NSCLC, OS and ORR were significantly greater for pembrolizumab independent of the dose compared with docetaxel (see Table 5.2).[10] Pembrolizumab benefited all patient subgroups except those with EGFR-mutant tumors and squamous histology, probably partly because of the small population size. Among the patients with at least 50% of tumor cells expressing PD-L1, pembrolizumab resulted in significantly longer PFS and OS than docetaxel, suggesting PD-L1 has value as a predictive biomarker.

Atezolizumab, a humanized IgG1 PD-L1 mAb, has also been approved for this indication, for tumors that express PD-L1, based on the POPLAR, FIR and BIRCH studies.[11,12] In the POPLAR study, atezolizumab was compared with docetaxel in 287 patients with pretreated NSCLC. PFS and ORR were similar in both groups but there was an OS benefit (see Table 5.2). OS, PFS and ORR tended to show increased atezolizumab benefit with increasing PD-L1 expression.[11] The benefit of atezolizumab was independent of histological subtype and tobacco history use. The ongoing OAK study will validate the efficacy of atezolizumab in patients with pretreated advanced NSCLC independently of PD-L1 positivity in tumor tissue.

Durvalumab, a humanized IgG1 PD-L1 mAb, is much earlier on in its clinical development, with early phase studies demonstrating a safety profile and excellent response rates that were durable.

Administration, efficacy and tolerability. No obvious features make one drug stand out from the others. Pembrolizumab and atezolizumab have a longer half life and are therefore administered every 3 weeks, whereas nivolumab has a shorter half life and is administered every 2 weeks when dosed at ≤ 3 mg/kg.

Safety, tolerability and efficacy appear to be similar across all PD-1 and PD-L1 inhibitors; about 10% of patients experience grade 3–4 adverse events. The most common adverse events tend to be fatigue, decreased appetite, nausea, rash and diarrhea. Immune-related adverse events are a concern, as they can occur idiosyncratically, unlike chemotherapy toxicity. Using KEYNOTE-010 as an example, about 20% of patients experienced immune-related adverse events; the most common were hyperthyroidism (4–6%), hypothyroidism (8%) and pneumonitis (4–5%). Grade 3–5 immune-related adverse events in 1% or more of patients were pneumonitis (2%) and severe skin reactions (1–2%).[10]

First-line monotherapy in NSCLC

In addition to the data in treatment-naive patients generated from phase I expanded cohorts, there are now specific first-line monotherapy studies. These randomized phase III studies are comparing PD-1/PD-L1 inhibitors alone with current platinum-based combination chemotherapy regimens, as summarized in Table 5.3.

Adjuvant and neoadjuvant studies

Given the efficacy already seen with these drugs in advanced NSCLC, several adjuvant and neoadjvuant studies are under way (Table 5.4). This is probably the best situation in which to demonstrate that an immunotherapy can cure more patients.

Combination therapy with chemotherapy

First-line platinum-based doublet chemotherapy is the standard of care for patients with advanced NSCLC who do not have a driver mutation, with a response rate of about 30% and a median OS of 8–10 months (see Chapter 6).

Early data show impressive response rates, ranging from 33% to 55% in CHECKMATE-012, 30% to 58% in KEYNOTE-021, and

TABLE 5.3

Clinical trials of first-line monotherapy studies with PD-1/PD-L1 inhibitors in advanced NSCLC

Trial (reference)	Drug	Population
CHECKMATE-026 (NCT02041533)	Nivolumab vs investigator choice of platinum-based combination chemotherapy	Enriched for PD-L1-positive patients
KEYNOTE-024 (NCT02142738)	Pembrolizumab vs investigator choice of platinum-based combination chemotherapy	PD-L1 positive (≥ 50%)
KEYNOTE-042 (NCT02220894)	Pembrolizumab vs investigator choice of platinum-based combination chemotherapy	Asia PD-L1 positive (1–49% vs ≥ 50%)
IMpower110 (NCT02409342)	Atezolizumab vs pemetrexed–platinum doublet chemotherapy	Non-squamous histology
IMpower111 (NCT02409355)	Atezolizumab vs gemcitabine–platinum doublet chemotherapy	Squamous histology
NEPTUNE (NCT02542293)	Durvalumab + tremelimumab vs investigator choice of platinum-based combination chemotherapy	
MYSTIC (NCT02453282)	Durvalumab +/- tremelimumab vs investigator choice of platinum-based combination chemotherapy	

PD-1, programmed cell death protein 1; PD-L1, programmed cell death ligand-1.

67% in early-phase atezolizumab studies. The concern with combining these therapies is toxicity, with reports of grade 3–4 adverse events ranging from 27% (KEYNOTE-021) to 45% (CHECKMATE-012). While the response rates are certainly high with these combinations,

TABLE 5.4

Adjuvant and neoadjuvant clinical trials in early stage NSCLC

Trial	Drug	Population	Study design	Reference
ANVIL	Nivolumab vs placebo after standard chemotherapy	Adjuvant therapy for resected early stage NSCLC	Open-label, phase III, randomized controlled trial	NCT02595944
KEYNOTE-091 (PEARLS)	Pembrolizumab vs placebo after standard chemotherapy for resected NSCLC	Adjuvant therapy for resected early stage NSCLC	Double-blind, phase III, randomized controlled trial	NCT02504372
Adjuvant atezolizumab	Atezolizumab vs best supportive care, after cisplatin-based standard chemotherapy	Adjuvant treatment for NSCLC	Open-label, phase III, randomized controlled trial	NCT02486718
Adjuvant durvalumab	Durvalumab vs placebo after standard adjuvant therapy	Adjuvant treatment for NSCLC	Double-blind, phase III, randomized controlled trial	NCT02273375
Adjuvant and neoadjuvant durvalumab	Durvalumab following neoadjuvant chemotherapy and adjuvant treatment for resectable stage IIIA (N2 disease) NSCLC	Neoadjuvant and adjuvant treatment for resectable stage IIIA (N2 disease) NSCLC	Single-arm phase II clinical trial	NCT02572843

the toxicities also appear to be increased. Mature follow-up data are required on safety and survival from these ongoing studies.

Combination therapy with other checkpoint inhibition

CTLA-4 antagonists have been developed in melanoma, but do not as yet have a role in the management of NSCLC. Furthermore, there is no reliable biomarker that predicts for response to CTLA-4 antagonism. However, there is potential for synergism by combining CTLA-4 inhibition with blockade of the PD-1/PD-L1 axis. Toxicity is a concern given the immune-related adverse events that have been seen with CTLA-4 antagonists.

Following CHECKMATE 012, a tolerable schedule of nivolumab plus ipilimumab is the focus of a phase III clinical trial (CHECKMATE 227) in chemotherapy-naive patients with advanced NSCLC.[13] KEYNOTE-021 combined pembrolizumab with ipilimumab in a dose escalation study in patients already treated with platinum chemotherapy. Interim data reported responses at all dose levels in 11 patients treated for 6 weeks or more, including one complete response. The data suggest that the combination has acceptable toxicity and robust responses.[14] Similar results have been seen with the combination of durvalumab and tremelimumab,[15] including in patients with PD-L1-negative disease; several combination studies are ongoing.

Combination therapy with small molecule inhibitors

A combination of drugs that target the PD-1/PD-L1 axis and personalized therapies for patients with NSCLC driver mutations (*EGFR* mutation and anaplastic lymphoma kinase [*ALK*] gene rearrangement; see Chapter 8) looks promising, as both *EGFR* mutations and *ALK* gene rearrangements upregulate PD-L1 expression via the MEK-ERK and PI3K-AKT pathways in vitro. This would suggest that oncogenic drivers induce immune escape in NSCLC through PD-L1 upregulation.

Preclinical and early phase clinical data from KEYNOTE-001 suggest that prior therapy with EGFR inhibitors is associated with a lack of response to PD-1 inhibition.

Several early phase clinical trials are looking at the combination of PD-1/PD-L1 checkpoint inhibition and EGFR inhibitors (e.g. KEYNOTE-021), EML4-ALK inhibitors (e.g. NCT02013219), MEK inhibitors (e.g. NCT02143466) and cMET inhibitors (e.g. NCT02323126). From early results, the combination of PD-1/PD-L1 inhibition and EGFR inhibition appears to be safe, as suggested by the results from the combination of gefitinib and durvalumab. However, efficacy data are still awaited.

Combination therapy with radiotherapy

Radiotherapy to a cancer may act as an antigen-releasing agent. Preclinical data and case reports suggest robust clinical responses in metastatic NSCLC and the potential for an abscopal effect.[16,17]

In advanced stage disease, studies are looking at palliative radiotherapy to a thoracic lesion (PEAR), while others are looking at the safety of stereotactic radiotherapy (Netherlands). For patients with locally advanced disease, durvalumab is being tested as a maintenance therapy after radical chemoradiotherapy (PACIFIC), while pembrolizumab is being assessed as a radiosensitizer with radical chemoradiotherapy (PARIS).

Key points – immuno-oncology

- Nivolumab should be considered as a second-line treatment option for patients with non-squamous cell histology whose tumors are positive for programmed cell death ligand-1 (PD-L1) and all patients with squamous cell histology.
- Pembrolizumab should be considered as a treatment option for all patients whose tumors are PD-L1 positive.
- Generally, programmed cell death protein-1 (PD-1) and PD-L1 inhibitors have a similar side-effect profile and efficacy.
- Combination strategies with both cytotoxic T-lymphoma-associated protein 4 (CTLA-4) antagonism and first-line chemotherapy offer better response rates; however, caution needs to be exercised with the inherent risk of increased toxicity.
- Strong PD-L1 staining is a biomarker for response to PD-1/PD-L1 inhibition.

References

1. Leach DR, Krummel MF, Allison JP. Enhancement of antitumor immunity by CTLA-4 blockade. *Science* 1996;271:1734–6.

2. Jing W, Li M, Zhang Y et al. PD-1/PD-L1 blockades in non-small-cell lung cancer therapy. *OncoTargets Ther* 2016;9:489–502.

3. Dai S, Jia R, Zhang X et al. The PD-1/PD-Ls pathway and autoimmune diseases. *Cell Immunol* 2014;290:72–9.

4. Brahmer J. Immune checkpoint blockade: the hope for immunotherapy as a treatment of lung cancer? *Semin Oncol* 2014;41:126–32.

5. Wu P, Wu D, Li L et al. PD-L1 and survival in solid tumors: a meta-analysis. *PLoS ONE* 2015;10:e0131403.

6. Wang A, Wang HY, Liu Y et al. The prognostic value of PD-L1 expression for non-small cell lung cancer patients: a meta-analysis. *Eur J Surg Oncol* 2015;41:450–6.

7. Brahmer J, Reckamp KL, Baas P et al. Nivolumab versus docetaxel in advanced squamous-cell non-small-cell lung cancer. *N Engl J Med* 2015; 373:123–35. CHECKMATE-017

8. Borghaei H, Paz-Ares L, Horn L et al. Nivolumab versus docetaxel in advanced nonsquamous non–small-cell lung cancer. *N Engl J Med* 2015; 373:1627–39. CHECKMATE-057

9. Garon EB, Rizvi NA, Hui R et al. Pembrolizumab for the treatment of non-small-cell lung cancer. *N Engl J Med* 2015;372:2018–28. KEYNOTE-001

10. Herbst RS, Baas P, Kim DW et al. Pembrolizumab versus docetaxel for previously treated, PD-L1-positive, advanced non-small-cell lung cancer (KEYNOTE-010): a randomised controlled trial. *Lancet Oncol* 2016;387:1540–50.

11. Fehrenbacher L, Spira A, Ballinger M et al. Atezolizumab versus docetaxel for patients with previously treated non-small-cell lung cancer (POPLAR): a multicentre, open-label, phase 2 randomised controlled trial. *Lancet* 2016;387:1837–46.

12. Besse B, Johnson M, Janne P et al. Phase II, single-arm trial (BIRCH) of atezolizumab as first-line or subsequent therapy for locally advanced or metastatic PD-L1-selected non-small cell lung cancer (NSCLC). *Ann Oncol* 2015;26(suppl 6):abstr. 16LBA.

13. Rizvi NA, Gettinger SN, Goldman JW et al. Safety and efficacy of first-line nivolumab (NIVO; anti-programmed death-1 [PD-1]) and ipilimumab in non-small cell lung cancer (NSCLC). *J Thorac Oncol* 2015;10:S176(abstr. 786).

14. Patnaik A, Socinski MA, Gubens MA et al. Phase 1 study of pembrolizumab (pembro; MK-3475) plus ipilimumab (IPI) as second-line therapy for advanced non-small cell lung cancer (NSCLC): KEYNOTE-021 cohort D. *J Clin Oncol* 2015; 33(suppl; abstr 8011).

15. Antonia S, Goldberg SB, Balmanoukian A et al. Safety and antitumour activity of durvalumab plus tremelimumab in non-small cell lung cancer: a multicentre, phase 1b study. *Lancet Oncol* 2016;17: 299–308.

16. Daly ME, Monjazeb AM, Kelly K. Clinical trials integrating immunotherapy and radiation for non-small-cell lung cancar. *J Thorac Oncol* 2015;10:1685–93.

17. Sharabi AB, Lim M, DeWeese TL, Drake CG. Radiation and checkpoint blockade immunotherapy: radiosensitisation and potential mechanisms of synergy. *Lancet Oncol* 2015;16:e498–509.

6 First and second-line chemotherapy in advanced NSCLC

Maria-Virginia Bluthgen MD, *Department of Cancer Medicine, Gustave Roussy, Villejuif, France*

Chemotherapy is still the mainstay of systemic treatment for patients with metastatic non-small-cell lung cancer (NSCLC). The main factors influencing chemotherapy regimen selection are histology of the tumor, comorbidities and performance status (PS). Since 2004, patients with tumors harboring sensitizing mutations in the epidermal growth factor receptor (*EGFR*) gene, may receive an EGFR tyrosine kinase inhibitor (TKI) as an alternative to chemotherapy (see Chapter 8). This chapter describes treatment for patients without such actionable mutations.

First-line chemotherapy

A systematic review showed that platinum-based therapy was associated with greater 1-year survival (RR 1.08, 95% CI 1.01–1.16) and increased response rate (RR 1.11, 95% CI 1.02–1.21) than non-platinum-based therapy.[1] The use of a platinum-based combination is the backbone of first-line treatment in patients with advanced NSCLC.

Cisplatin- and carboplatin-based regimens yield similar improvements in survival but with different toxicity profiles; cisplatin-based chemotherapy is associated with more severe nephrotoxicity, nausea and vomiting.[2–4] However, some trials suggest that cisplatin may achieve higher response rates and survival outcomes. Comorbidities, clinical presentation (determining need of response) and toxicity profile, are all factors that may influence the selection of the preferred platinum compound for an individual patient.

In randomized controlled trials of patients with advanced disease and good PS, cisplatin-based chemotherapy has shown a significant improvement over best supportive care (BSC) in terms of disease progression, survival and palliation of disease-related symptoms.[5,6] Furthermore, a meta-analysis of randomized trials observed that a two-drug regimen significantly increased tumor response (OR 0.42,

CI 95% 0.37–0.47, p<0.001) and 1-year survival (OR 0.80, CI 95% 0.70–0.91, p<0.001) compared with single-agent treatment, although there was a significant increase in adverse events.[7]

Two-drug combinations comprised of a platinum and a cytotoxic agent, such as gemcitabine, vinorelbine, docetaxel or paclitaxel, have all resulted in similar survival.[8–10] However, toxicity profiles may differ. Differences in survival outcomes have been reported depending on the histology of NSCLC. For example, the benefit of pemetrexed appears to be restricted to non-squamous tumors.[11]

Three-(cytotoxic)-drug combinations do not give superior survival at 1 year (OR 1.01, 95% CI 0.85–1.21, p=0.88) over two-drug combinations, but do significantly increase the number of toxic events.[7]

Combinations with targeted therapy are an alternative option for first-line systemic treatment in selected patients. Two randomized trials have evaluated the efficacy of bevacizumab, a monoclonal antibody targeting vascular endothelial growth factor (VEGF), added to standard first-line platinum-based combination chemotherapy.[12,13] Both trials showed benefit in terms of progression-free survival (PFS) in patients who received the antiangiogenic therapy, but a significant difference in overall survival (OS) was only seen in those who received carboplatin–paclitaxel (12.3 vs 10.3 months; HR: 0.79 p=0.003 favoring bevacizumab). A significant bleeding rate of 4.4% was seen in the chemotherapy plus bevacizumab group compared with 0.7% in the chemotherapy only group.[12]

Two phase III trials have evaluated the addition of necitumumab, a recombinant antibody targeting EGFR, to a two-drug platinum combination in patients with squamous and non-squamous lung cancer.[14,15] Median OS was prolonged by a modest amount with the combination of the target therapy and cisplatin–gemcitabine in the squamous cell population.[14]

No other target agents have demonstrated clinically meaningful survival improvement in first-line treatment.[16,17]

Chemotherapy in the elderly

The survival benefit in fit, elderly patients with NSCLC receiving platinum-based combination treatment appears to be similar to that seen in younger patients.[18] A survival benefit was demonstrated in patients aged 70–89 years who received a weekly carboplatin–paclitaxel combination compared with a single-agent regimen, despite an increased but manageable toxicity profile.[19] Non-platinum-based combinations have not demonstrated a survival benefit over single agents in this population.[20]

Some series and prospective trials have shown survival benefit and improved symptom control with combinations compared with single agents in the elderly with PS2, although the benefit was much lower than that seen in patients with PS 0–1.[21,22]

Duration of chemotherapy

Historically, continuation of cytotoxic chemotherapy combinations with the same two drugs for more than 4 cycles has shown no survival advantage but has increased related toxicities. However, these studies were done before the use of well-tolerated drugs like pemetrexed, which has now been evaluated as both a first-line combination therapy and a maintenance single agent.

Maintenance therapy

The two strategies for maintenance therapy following disease control after first-line treatment are continuous and switch maintenance.

Continuous maintenance with pemetrexed has demonstrated statistical improvement in OS in patients with NSCLC compared with placebo (HR 0.78, 95% CI 0.64–0.96, $p=0.0195$; median OS 13.9 vs 11 months).[23] A benefit in PFS only was seen with the same strategy in combination with gemcitabine.[24]

Switch maintenance with pemetrexed after non-progression following a non-pemetrexed combination regimen, has also shown a benefit in terms of PFS and OS in one randomized trial.[25] Collectively, these data suggest that survival could be improved with maintenance pemetrexed for patients with non-squamous histology.

Second-line chemotherapy

Almost all patients will eventually progress after first-line treatment and will require further treatment. Factors to take into account when choosing further therapy include PS, previous treatment, histology and whether a driver mutation is present.

Two chemotherapy drugs are currently approved for second-line treatment of advanced NSCLC: docetaxel and pemetrexed. In 1999, a significant survival benefit (37% vs 11%) and improvement in disease-related symptoms was demonstrated with second-line docetaxel compared with BSC in patients with advanced NSCLC and good PS who had relapsed following a first-line platinum-based treatment.[26] In 2004, second-line pemetrexed showed equivalent efficacy with fewer side effects to docetaxel.[27]

While combinations of cytotoxic drugs have been successful in improving efficacy compared with single agents in the first-line setting, the role of second-line combination therapy is less clear.[28] Several randomized studies have been performed in patients with NSCLC comparing second-line docetaxel-based combination chemotherapy with docetaxel single agent: no significant differences in response rate, median survival or PFS were reported.[29-33] In two randomized phase II trials, pemetrexed-based combination therapy produced a higher response rate than the single agent but showed no benefit in terms of survival.[34] Two meta-analyses addressing the efficacy of combined therapy found no difference in OS between the two strategies, but a statistically significant increase in PFS (14 vs 11 weeks; HR=0.79, p=0.0009) and response rate (15.1% vs 7.3%, p=0.0004) in favor of the combination therapy, albeit with a much higher incidence of adverse events.[35,36]

Re-challenge with platinum-based regimens is a widely used strategy in ovarian and small-cell lung cancer with major benefit reported in patients relapsing after 6 months or more.[37,38] To date, no prospective phase III studies directly addressing this approach have been conducted in patients with NSCLC, but this strategy is reasonable in clinical practice.

Second-line cytotoxic chemotherapy combined with a targeted agent has also shown promising results. Ramucirumab, a novel antiangiogenic IgG1 antibody that targets the extracellular domain of VEGF receptor-2 (VEGFR2), has been evaluated in combination with conventional docetaxel therapy versus docetaxel plus placebo in the REVEL trial. The results showed prolonged OS (10.5 vs 9.1 months;

HR=0.86, p=0.023) and PFS (4.5 vs 3.0 months; HR=0.76, p<0.0001) in the ramucirumab group.[39]

The addition of nintedanib, an oral inhibitor of *VEGFR1–3/FGFR1–3/PDGFR/RET/FLT3/Src*, to conventional docetaxel therapy has been tested in 1314 patients. Results demonstrated a significant improvement in PFS (3.5 vs 2.7 months; HR=0.85, p=0.007) in all predefined subgroups. OS was significantly longer among patients with adenocarcinoma histology (12.6 vs 10.3 months; HR=0.83, p=0.0359) and the drug has been approved by the European Medicines Agency for this indication.[40]

Key points – first- and second-line chemotherapy in advanced NSCLC

- Treatment for patients with metastatic NSCLC without an actional somatic gene mutation consists of systemic chemotherapy; regimen selection is based on histology, comorbidities and performance status (PS).
- Platinum-based combinations are the backbone of first-line treatment for patients with advanced NSCLC.
- Pemetrexed regimens are restricted to non-squamous histology.
- Pemetrexed as continuous or switch maintenance prolongs survival over no maintenance in patients with non-squamous histologies and PS 0,1.
- Bevacizumab combined with a paclitaxel regimen can provide a survival benefit over a paclitaxel regimen alone in patients with non-squamous subgroups.
- Advanced age alone should not preclude appropriate NSCLC treatment.
- Two chemotherapy drugs have been approved for the treatment of advanced NSCLC in the second-line setting: docetaxel and pemetrexed.
- Platinum re-challenge could represent a potential option for fit, relapsed patients with a platinum-free interval treatment of more than 6 months.

References

1. Rajeswaran A, Trojan A, Burnand B, Giannelli M. Efficacy and side effects of cisplatin- and carboplatin-based doublet chemotherapeutic regimens versus non-platinum-based doublet chemotherapeutic regimens as first line treatment of metastatic non-small-cell lung carcinoma: a systematic review of randomized controlled trials. *Lung Cancer* 2008;59:1–11.

2. Jiang J, Liang X, Zhou X et al. A meta-analysis of randomized controlled trials comparing carboplatin-based to cisplatin-based chemotherapy in advanced non-small cell lung cancer. *Lung Cancer* 2007;57:348–58.

3. Hotta K. Meta-analysis of randomized clinical trials comparing cisplatin to carboplatin in patients with advanced non-small-cell lung cancer. *J Clin Oncol* 2004;22:3852–9.

4. Ardizzoni A, Boni L, Tiseo M et al. Cisplatin- versus carboplatin-based chemotherapy in first-line treatment of advanced non-small-cell lung cancer: an individual patient data meta-analysis. *JNCI J Natl Cancer Inst* 2007;99:847–57.

5. Spiro SG. Chemotherapy versus supportive care in advanced non-small cell lung cancer: improved survival without detriment to quality of life. *Thorax* 2004;59:828–36.

6. Zhong C, Liu H, Jiang L et al. Chemotherapy plus best supportive care versus best supportive care in patients with non-small cell lung cancer: a meta-analysis of randomized controlled trials. *PLoS ONE* 2013;8:e58466.

7. Delbaldo C, Michiels S, Rolland E et al. Second or third additional chemotherapy drug for non-small cell lung cancer in patients with advanced disease. *Cochrane Database Syst Rev* 2012;(4): CD004569.

8. Weick JK, Crowley J, Natale RB et al. A randomized trial of five cisplatin-containing treatments in patients with metastatic non-small-cell lung cancer: a Southwest Oncology Group study. *J Clin Oncol* 1991;9:1157–62.

9. Douillard JY, Laporte S, Fossella F et al. Comparison of docetaxel- and vinca alkaloid-based chemotherapy in the first-line treatment of advanced non-small cell lung cancer: a meta-analysis of seven randomized clinical trials. *J Thorac Oncol* 2007;2:939–46.

10. Schiller JH, Harrington D, Belani CP et al. Comparison of four chemotherapy regimens for advanced non-small-cell lung cancer. *N Engl J Med* 2002;346:92–8.

11. Besse B, Adjei A, Baas P et al. 2nd ESMO Consensus Conference on Lung Cancer: non-small-cell lung cancer first-line/second and further lines of treatment in advanced disease. *Ann Oncol* 2014;25:1475–84.

12. Sandler A, Gray R, Perry MC et al. Paclitaxel–carboplatin alone or with bevacizumab for non-small-cell lung cancer. N Engl J Med 2006;355:2542–50.

13. Reck M, von Pawel J, Zatloukal P et al. Phase III trial of cisplatin plus gemcitabine with either placebo or bevacizumab as first-line therapy for nonsquamous non-small-cell lung cancer: AVAiL. J Clin Oncol 2009;27:1227–34.

14. Thatcher N, Hirsch FR, Luft AV et al. Necitumumab plus gemcitabine and cisplatin versus gemcitabine and cisplatin alone as first-line therapy in patients with stage IV squamous non-small-cell lung cancer (SQUIRE): an open-label, randomised, controlled phase 3 trial. Lancet Oncol 2015;16:763–74.

15. Paz-Ares L, Mezger J, Ciuleanu TE et al. Necitumumab plus pemetrexed and cisplatin as first-line therapy in patients with stage IV non-squamous non-small-cell lung cancer (INSPIRE): an open-label, randomised, controlled phase 3 study. Lancet Oncol 2015;16: 328–37.

16. Pirker R, Pereira JR, Szczesna A et al. Cetuximab plus chemotherapy in patients with advanced non-small-cell lung cancer (FLEX): an open-label randomised phase III trial. Lancet 2009;373:1525–31.

17. Lynch TJ, Patel T, Dreisbach L et al. Cetuximab and first-line taxane/carboplatin chemotherapy in advanced non-small-cell lung cancer: results of the randomized multicenter phase III trial BMS099. J Clin Oncol 2010;28:911–17.

18. Langer CJ, Manola J, Bernardo P et al. Cisplatin-based therapy for elderly patients with advanced non-small-cell lung cancer: implications of Eastern Cooperative Oncology Group 5592, a randomized trial. J Natl Cancer Inst 2002;94:173–81.

19. Quoix E, Zalcman G, Oster JP et al. Carboplatin and weekly paclitaxel doublet chemotherapy compared with monotherapy in elderly patients with advanced non-small-cell lung cancer: IFCT-0501 randomised, phase 3 trial. Lancet 2011;378:1079–88.

20. Gridelli C, Perrone F, Gallo C et al. Chemotherapy for elderly patients with advanced non-small-cell lung cancer: the Multicenter Italian Lung Cancer in the Elderly Study (MILES) phase III randomized trial. J Nat Cancer Inst 2003;95:362–72.

21. Zukin M, Barrios CH, Rodrigues Pereira J et al. Randomized phase III trial of single-agent pemetrexed versus carboplatin and pemetrexed in patients with advanced non-small-cell lung cancer and Eastern Cooperative Oncology Group performance status of 2. J Clin Oncol 2013;31:2849–53.

22. Lilenbaum RC, Herndon II JE, List MA et al. Single-agent versus combination chemotherapy in advanced non-small-cell lung cancer: The Cancer and Leukemia Group B (study 9730). *J Clin Oncol* 2005;23:190–6.

23. Paz-Ares LG, de Marinis F, Dediu M et al. PARAMOUNT: final overall survival results of the phase III study of maintenance pemetrexed versus placebo immediately after induction treatment with pemetrexed plus cisplatin for advanced nonsquamous non-small-cell lung cancer. *J Clin Oncol* 2013;31:2895–902.

24. Brodowicz T, Krzakowski M, Zwitter M et al. Cisplatin and gemcitabine first-line chemotherapy followed by maintenance gemcitabine or best supportive care in advanced non-small cell lung cancer: a phase III trial. *Lung Cancer* 2006;52:155–63.

25. Ciuleanu, T, Brodowicz, T, Zielinski C et al. Maintenance pemetrexed plus best supportive care versus placebo plus best supportive care for non-small-cell lung cancer: a randomised, double-blind, phase 3 study. *Lancet* 2009;374:1432–40.

26. Shepherd FA, Dancey J, Ramlau R et al. Prospective randomized trial of docetaxel versus best supportive care in patients with non-small-cell lung cancer previously treated with platinum-based chemotherapy. *J Clin Oncol* 2000;18:2095–103.

27. Hanna N, Shepherd FA, Fossella FV et al. Randomized phase III trial of pemetrexed versus docetaxel in patients with non-small-cell lung cancer previously treated with chemotherapy. *J Clin Oncol* 2004;22:1589–97.

28. Bluthgen M-V, Besse B. Second-line combination therapies in nonsmall cell lung cancer without known driver mutations. *Eur Respir Rev* 2015;24:582–93.

29. Takeda K, Negoro S, Tamura T et al. Phase III trial of docetaxel plus gemcitabine versus docetaxel in second-line treatment for non-small-cell lung cancer: results of a Japan Clinical Oncology Group trial (JCOG0104). *Ann Oncol* 2009;20:835–41.

30. Gebbia V, Gridelli C, Verusio C et al. Weekly docetaxel vs. docetaxel-based combination chemotherapy as second-line treatment of advanced non-small-cell lung cancer patients. The DISTAL-2 randomized trial. *Lung Cancer* 2009;63:251–8.

31. Pallis AG, Agelaki S, Agelidou A et al. A randomized phase III study of the docetaxel/carboplatin combination versus docetaxel single-agent as second line treatment for patients with advanced/metastatic non-small cell lung cancer. *BMC Cancer* 2010;10:633.

32. Pectasides D, Pectasides M, Farmakis D et al. Comparison of docetaxel and docetaxel–irinotecan combination as second-line chemotherapy in advanced non-small-cell lung cancer: a randomized phase II trial. *Ann Oncol* 2005;16:294–9.

33. Wachters FM, Groen HJM, Biesma B et al. A randomised phase II trial of docetaxel vs docetaxel and irinotecan in patients with stage IIIb–IV non-small-cell lung cancer who failed first-line treatment. *Br J Cancer* 2005;92:15–20.

34. Ardizzoni A, Tiseo M, Boni L et al. Pemetrexed versus pemetrexed and carboplatin as second-line chemotherapy in advanced non-small-cell lung cancer: results of the GOIRC 02-2006 randomized phase II study and pooled analysis with the NVALT7 trial. *J Clin Oncol* 2012;30:4501–7.

35. Di Maio M, Chiodini P, Georgoulias V et al. Meta-analysis of single-agent chemotherapy compared with combination chemotherapy as second-line treatment of advanced non-small-cell lung cancer. *J Clin Oncol* 2009;27:1836–43.

36. Qi WX, Shen Z, Yao Y. Meta-analysis of docetaxel-based doublet versus docetaxel alone as second-line treatment for advanced non-small-cell lung cancer. *Cancer Chemother Pharmacol* 2012;69:99–106.

37. Parmar MK, Ledermann JA, Colombo N et al. Paclitaxel plus platinum-based chemotherapy versus conventional platinum-based chemotherapy in women with relapsed ovarian cancer: the ICON4/AGO-OVAR-2.2 trial. *Lancet* 2003;361:2099–106.

38. Genestreti G, Metro G, Kenmotsu H et al. Final outcome results of platinum-sensitive small cell lung cancer (SCLC) patients treated with platinum-based chemotherapy rechallenge: a multi-institutional retrospective analysis. *J Clin Oncol* 2014; 32(suppl; abstr. 7600).

39. Garon EB, Ciuleanu TE, Arrieta O et al. Ramucirumab plus docetaxel versus placebo plus docetaxel for second-line treatment of stage IV non-small-cell lung cancer after disease progression on platinum-based therapy (REVEL): a multicentre, double-blind, randomised phase 3 trial. *Lancet* 2014;384:665–73.

40. Reck M, Kaiser R, Mellemgaard A et al. Docetaxel plus nintedanib versus docetaxel plus placebo in patients with previously treated non-small-cell lung cancer (LUME-Lung 1): a phase 3, double-blind, randomised controlled trial. *Lancet Oncol* 2014;15:143–55.

Gokoulakrichenane Loganadane MD *and Antonin Levy* MD,
Department of Radiation Oncology, Thoracic Oncology Institute,
Gustave Roussy Cancer Campus, Villejuif, France

Brain metastases (BM) are common in the natural history of non-small-cell lung cancer (NSCLC) and, with advances in imaging modalities and improvements in systemic disease control, both the incidence and prevalence of BM are rising. BM have deleterious effects on many critical neurological functions. Survival ranges from 3 to 14.8 months, depending on the lung diagnosis-specific graded prognostic assessment (DS-GPA): age, Karnofsky Performance Score (KPS), presence of extracranial metastases (ECM) and number of BM (Table 7.1).[1,2] The

TABLE 7.1

Diagnosis-Specific Graded Prognostic Assessment (DS-GPA) for brain metastases from lung cancer[2]

	GPA scoring criteria		
	0	0.5	1.0
Age (years)	> 60	50–60	< 50
KPS	< 70	70–80	90–100
ECM	+	n/a	–
No. of BM	> 3	2–3	1

Total score = _____

Total score	Median survival time (months)
0–1.0	3.02 (2.62–3.84)
1.5–2.0	5.49 (4.83–6.40)
2.5–3.0	9.43 (8.38–10.80)
3.5–4.0	14.78 (11.80–18.80)

BM, brain metastases; ECM, extracranial metastases; KPS, Karnofsky Performance Score.

DS-GPA score has a central role in the management of patients; focal interventions should preferentially be delivered to patients with a good prognosis. Radiation therapy, surgery and systemic therapies are options for the management of metastatic lesions in the brain.

Diagnosis

Common symptoms include headache, neurological deficit and seizures. Although differential diagnoses such as abscess or stroke must be considered, new neurological symptoms should be assumed to be related to the known cancer until proven otherwise.

CT or MRI of the brain is used to confirm the diagnosis. MRI is preferable to CT because of its higher resolution and ability to find smaller and solitary lesions. BM typically appear as contrast-enhanced lesions on CT or MRI (sequence T1 with gadolinium). T2-weighted or FLAIR (fluid-attenuated inversion recovery) images may show edema around the tumor.

Treatment options

An algorithm for the management of BM is shown in Figure 1.[2]

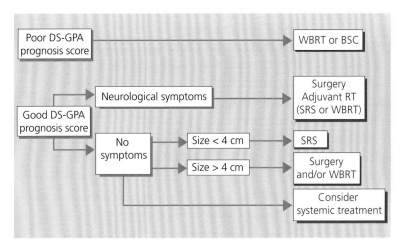

Figure 7.1 Proposed algorithm for the management of brain metastases. BSC, best supportive care; DS-GPA, Diagnosis-Specific Graded Prognostic Assessment (score) (see Table 7.1); RT, radiotherapy; SRS, stereotactic radiosurgery; WBRT, whole brain radiotherapy.

Surgery. Urgent surgery is considered when a tumor causes significant edema and mass effect with consequent hydrocephalus or herniation. The presence of a single metastatic brain lesion also needs discussion at a multidisciplinary meeting attended by a neurosurgeon. In small randomized trials in patients with a single metastatic brain lesion, surgery plus whole brain radiotherapy (WBRT) increased survival compared with WBRT alone.[3,4] Conversely, in another small randomized trial, no survival benefit was demonstrated.[5] Nowadays, surgery followed by stereotactic radiosurgery (SRS) to the tumor bed is an option. SRS decreases the likelihood of local relapse after resection.[6] However, it appears to be associated with an increased risk of leptomeningeal relapse and radionecrosis.[7] A randomized phase III trial is currently comparing adjuvant WBRT with SRS.[8]

No randomized trials have addressed the role of surgery for multiple lesions, and retrospective data are conflicting. As 7–10% of patients who undergo surgery suffer from major complications, candidates should be selected cautiously.[9]

Radiotherapy

Whole brain radiation therapy continues to be the standard of care for patients with a poor prognosis according to the DS-GPA (i.e. patients who are not candidates for surgery or SRS) with multiple (more than 3–5) BM. The most widely used schedule is 30 Gy over 2 weeks (10 daily fractions). WBRT does not increase survival or quality of life compared with best supportive care (BSC), as reported in the large prospective randomized Quartz trial.[10]

Well-established acute side effects of WBRT, which are not typically associated with SRS (see below), include alopecia, dermatitis and asthenia. The main drawbacks are a decline in neurocognitive function in long-term survivors and a negative effect on quality of life. It should be mentioned that tumor progression also affects neurocognitive function, which can make the assessement of WBRT difficult.[11] Strategies to overcome neurocognitive impairment after WBRT include hippocampus-sparing WBRT[12] or neuroprotective agents. Concurrent memantine, an oral N-methyl-D-aspartate (NMDA) receptor antagonist, was found to delay time to cognitive decline, but only

29% of the patients (n=149) were available for assessment of the primary endpoint, memory decline, at 24 weeks.[13]

Stereotactic radiosurgery concentrates high-dose ablative radiation within a tumor while avoiding radiation of the surrounding healthy tissue. It is suitable for small well-defined metastases (< 4 cm). Focal high-dose irradiation, compared with neurosurgery, has the ability to treat surgically inaccessible areas and several lesions at a time; furthermore, it is non-invasive and cost-effective. In a large randomized trial (RTOG 9508), an SRS boost increased survival in patients with a good prognostic score and a single lesion.[14,15] Although no randomized trials have directly compared surgery to SRS, SRS seems to provide a similar local control rate (80–90%), especially when SRS is combined with WBRT.

In a large trial conducted by the European Organization for Research and Treatment of Cancer (EORTC 22952-26001), the addition of WBRT significantly decreased local relapse (at the initial site and within the brain) but there was no significant difference in overall survival.[16]

The application of WBRT after SRS (or surgery) may have a negative effect on cognitive function.[17] Thus, SRS is now generally performed without WBRT in patients with a limited number of lesions (up to 3). SRS without WBRT is feasible as the initial treatment for patients with 5–10 BM.[18]

SRS leads to radiation necrosis in approximately 10% of patients, especially those who receive combined (WBRT+SRS) radiation.[19] It can be difficult to distinguish between radiation necrosis and recurrent BM on conventional MRI. Perfusion MRI sequences may be useful, as recurrent BM are characterized by increased vascular perfusion, while radiation necrosis has a decreased vascularity.[20]

Systemic therapies

Glucocorticoids improve symptoms in up to 75% of patients with cerebral edema and are indicated in patients with neurological symptoms. Dexamethasone is the glucocorticoid of choice because of its low mineralocorticoid effect and long half life.[21]

Chemotherapy. Several prospective trials have demonstrated the activity of first-line chemotherapy for NSCLC metastases, with responses rates of 23–50% for platinum-based regimens.[22–25] Intracerebral response rates were shown to correlate with systemic response, although intracranial response rates remain slighty inferior to overall response rate.

The order of chemotherapy and radiotherapy is often dictated by how symptomatic a patient is and their performance status (PS). Radiotherapy is often used for very symptomatic patients with poor PS. Systemic treatment is usually the first choice for asymptomatic or minimally symptomatic BM, particularly if a sensitizing driver mutation is present in the tumor. Concurrent WBRT and chemotherapy resulted in higher neurocognitive deficit without clear benefit in response rate or survival.[26,27] European Society Medical Oncology (ESMO) guidelines and data from randomized trials support chemotherapy as a reasonable first-line treatment option for patients with stage IV NSCLC and asymptomatic BM.[28–30] Chemotherapy may also be proposed as a salvage treatment.

Targeted therapies. A substantial percentage of patients have been found to have specific somatic genetic alterations underlying their tumors that can be targeted by specific molecular compounds (see Chapter 8). Epidermal growth factor receptor (EGFR) tyrosine kinase inhibitors (TKI) have antitumor activity in patients with NSCLC BM. Concurrent erlotinib and WBRT has demonstrated a good overall response rate (86%) with a median overall survival of 12 months.[31] In the randomized RTOG 0302 trial, which addressed the use of erlotinib (or temozolomide or no systemic treatment) with WBRT and SRS, toxicity was higher with systemic therapies than with WBRT/SRS alone.

A high incidence of BM is seen in patients who have NSCLC with anaplastic lymphoma kinase (*ALK*) rearrangement (40%).[32] Patients with BM from *ALK*-rearranged NSCLC who are treated with radiotherapy (SRS and/or WBRT) and crizotinib may have prolonged survival.[33] Newer *ALK*-driven targeted therapy also seems promising.[34–36] It is therefore reasonable to propose the use of targeted molecular compounds as first-line treatment for selected patients with stage IV NSCLC and asymptomatic BM.

The intracranial effect of immunotherapies has also been described.

Key points – management of brain metastases

- Brain metastases (BM) are common in the natural history of patients with NSCLC.
- The Diagnosis-Specific Graded Prognostic Assessment (DS-GPA) score, which is based on age, Karnofsky performance score, the presence of extracranial metastases and the number of BM, can guide clinicians' decisions.
- Surgical resection may be required for patients presenting with neurological symptoms or a large single lesion.
- Whole brain radiotherapy was the standard treatment for patients with a poor prognosis, but this has recently been challenged.
- Stereotactic radiosurgery could be given to patients with a limited number of small well-defined BM, as it provides excellent local control with limited toxicities.
- Systemic treatment (chemotherapy or targeted compounds) is a reasonable treatment option for asymptomatic patients.

References

1. Sperduto CM, Watanabe Y, Mullan J et al. A validation study of a new prognostic index for patients with brain metastases: the Graded Prognostic Assessment. *J Neurosurg* 2008;109 Suppl:87–9.

2. Sperduto PW, Kased N, Roberge D et al. Summary report on the graded prognostic assessment: an accurate and facile diagnosis-specific tool to estimate survival for patients with brain metastases. *J Clin Oncol* 2012;30:419–25.

3. Patchell RA, Tibbs PA, Walsh JW et al. A randomized trial of surgery in the treatment of single metastases to the brain. *N Engl J Med* 1990;322:494–500.

4. Noordijk EM, Vecht CJ, Haaxma-Reiche H et al. The choice of treatment of single brain metastasis should be based on extracranial tumor activity and age. *Int J Radiat Oncol Biol Phys* 1994;29:711–17.

5. Mintz AH, Kestle J, Rathbone MP et al. A randomized trial to assess the efficacy of surgery in addition to radiotherapy in patients with a single cerebral metastasis. *Cancer* 1996;78:1470–6.

6. Roberge D, Parney I, Brown PD. Radiosurgery to the postoperative surgical cavity: who needs evidence? *Int J Radiat Oncol Biol Phys* 2012;83:486–93.

7. Johnson MD, Avkshtol V, Baschnagel AM et al. Surgical Resection of brain metastases and the risk of leptomeningeal recurrence in patients treated with stereotactic radiosurgery. *Int J Radiat Oncol Biol Phys* 2016;94:537–43.

8. ClinicalTrials.gov. Stereotactic radiosurgery or whole-brain radiation therapy in treating patients with brain metastases that have been removed by surgery. https://clinicaltrials.gov/ct2/show/NCT01372774, last accessed 11 August 2016.

9. Patel AJ, Suki D, Hatiboglu MA et al. Impact of surgical methodology on the complication rate and functional outcome of patients with a single brain metastasis. *J Neurosurg* 2015;122:1132–43.

10. Mulvenna PM, Nankivell MG, Barton R et al. Whole brain radiotherapy for brain metastases from non-small cell lung cancer: quality of life (QoL) and overall survival (OS) results from the UK Medical Research Council QUARTZ randomised clinical trial (ISRCTN 3826061). *J Clin Oncol* 2015;33(suppl;abstr 8005).

11. Li J, Bentzen SM, Renschler M, Mehta MP. Regression after whole-brain radiation therapy for brain metastases correlates with survival and improved neurocognitive function. *J Clin Oncol* 2007;25:1260–6.

12. Gondi V, Pugh SL, Tome WA et al. Preservation of memory with conformal avoidance of the hippocampal neural stem-cell compartment during whole-brain radiotherapy for brain metastases (RTOG 0933): a phase II multi-institutional trial. *J Clin Oncol* 2014;32:3810–16.

13. Brown PD, Pugh S, Laack NN et al. Memantine for the prevention of cognitive dysfunction in patients receiving whole-brain radiotherapy: a randomized, double-blind, placebo-controlled trial. *Neuro Oncol* 2013;15:1429–37.

14. Andrews DW, Scott CB, Sperduto PW et al. Whole brain radiation therapy with or without stereotactic radiosurgery boost for patients with one to three brain metastases: phase III results of the RTOG 9508 randomised trial. *Lancet* 2004;363:1665–72.

15. Kondziolka D, Patel A, Lunsford LD et al. Stereotactic radiosurgery plus whole brain radiotherapy versus radiotherapy alone for patients with multiple brain metastases. *Int J Radiat Oncol Biol Phys* 1999;45:427–34.

16. Kocher M, Soffietti R, Abacioglu U et al. Adjuvant whole-brain radiotherapy versus observation after radiosurgery or surgical resection of one to three cerebral metastases: results of the EORTC 22952-26001 study. *J Clin Oncol* 2011;29:134–41.

17. Chang EL, Wefel JS, Hess KR et al. Neurocognition in patients with brain metastases treated with radiosurgery or radiosurgery plus whole-brain irradiation: a randomised controlled trial. *Lancet Oncol* 2009;10:1037–44.

18. Yamamoto M, Serizawa T, Shuto T et al. Stereotactic radiosurgery for patients with multiple brain metastases (JLGK0901): a multi-institutional prospective observational study. *Lancet Oncol* 2014;15:387–95.

19. Minniti G, Clarke E, Lanzetta G et al. Stereotactic radiosurgery for brain metastases: analysis of outcome and risk of brain radionecrosis. *Radiat Oncol* 2011;6:48.

20. Mitsuya K, Nakasu Y, Horiguchi S et al. Perfusion weighted magnetic resonance imaging to distinguish the recurrence of metastatic brain tumors from radiation necrosis after stereotactic radiosurgery. *J Neurooncol* 2010;99:81–8.

21. Vecht CJ, Hovestadt A, Verbiest HB et al. Dose-effect relationship of dexamethasone on Karnofsky performance in metastatic brain tumors: a randomized study of doses of 4, 8, and 16 mg per day. *Neurology* 1994;44:675–80.

22. Cotto C, Berille J, Souquet PJ et al. A phase II trial of fotemustine and cisplatin in central nervous system metastases from non-small cell lung cancer. *Eur J Cancer* 1996;32A:69–71.

23. Fujita A, Fukuoka S, Takabatake H et al. Combination chemotherapy of cisplatin, ifosfamide, and irinotecan with rhG-CSF support in patients with brain metastases from non-small cell lung cancer. *Oncology* 2000;59:291–5.

24. Besse B, Le Moulec S, Mazières J et al. Bevacizumab in patients with nonsquamous non-small cell lung cancer and asymptomatic, untreated brain metastases (BRAIN): a nonrandomized, phase II study. *Clin Cancer Res* 2015;21:1896–903.

25. Barlesi F, Gervais R, Lena H et al. Pemetrexed and cisplatin as first-line chemotherapy for advanced non-small-cell lung cancer (NSCLC) with asymptomatic inoperable brain metastases: a multicenter phase II trial (GFPC 07-01). *Ann Oncol* 2011;22:2466–70.

26. Verger E, Gil M, Yaya R, et al. Temozolomide and concomitant whole brain radiotherapy in patients with brain metastases: a phase II randomized trial. *Int J Radiat Oncol Biol Phys* 2005;61:185–91.

27. Soussain C, Ricard D, Fike JR et al. CNS complications of radiotherapy and chemotherapy. *Lancet* 2009;374:1639–51.

28. Peters S, Adjei AA, Gridelli C et al. Metastatic non-small-cell lung cancer (NSCLC): ESMO Clinical Practice Guidelines for diagnosis, treatment and follow-up. *Ann Oncol* 2012;23(Suppl 7):vii56–64.

29. Lee DH, Han J-Y, Kim HT et al. Primary chemotherapy for newly diagnosed nonsmall cell lung cancer patients with synchronous brain metastases compared with whole-brain radiotherapy administered first: result of a randomized pilot study. *Cancer* 2008;113:143–9.

30. Robinet G, Thomas P, Breton JL et al. Results of a phase III study of early versus delayed whole brain radiotherapy with concurrent cisplatin and vinorelbine combination in inoperable brain metastasis of non-small-cell lung cancer: Groupe Français de Pneumo-Cancérologie (GFPC) Protocol 95-1. *Ann Oncol* 2001;12:59–67.

31. Sperduto PW, Wang M, Robins HI et al. A phase 3 trial of whole brain radiation therapy and stereotactic radiosurgery alone versus WBRT and SRS with temozolomide or erlotinib for non-small cell lung cancer and 1 to 3 brain metastases: Radiation Therapy Oncology Group 0320. *Int J Radiat Oncol Biol Phys* 2013;85:1312–18.

32. Shaw AT, Kim D-W, Nakagawa K et al. Crizotinib versus chemotherapy in advanced *ALK*-positive lung cancer. *N Engl J Med* 2013;368:2385–94.

33. Kim DW, Mehra R, Tan DSW et al. Activity and safety of ceritinib in patients with *ALK*-rearranged non-small-cell lung cancer (ASCEND-1): updated results from the multicentre, open-label, phase 1 trial. *Lancet Oncol* 2016;17: 452–63.

34. Camidge DR, Bang Y-J, Kwak EL et al. Activity and safety of crizotinib in patients with *ALK*-positive non-small-cell lung cancer: updated results from a phase 1 study. *Lancet Oncol* 2012;13:1011–19.

35. Maillet D, Martel-Lafay I, Arpin D et al. Ineffectiveness of crizotinib on brain metastases in two cases of lung adenocarcinoma with *EML4-ALK* rearrangement. *J Thorac Oncol* 2013;8:e30–1.

36. Johung KL, Yeh N, Desai NB et al. Extended survival and prognostic factors for patients with *ALK*-rearranged non-small-cell lung cancer and brain metastasis. *J Clin Oncol* 2016;34:123–9.

Jordi Remon MD, *Medical Oncology Department, Gustave Roussy, Villejuif, France.*

The molecular profiling of advanced non-small-cell lung cancer (NSCLC) for known oncogenic drivers is a recommended part of routine care. This personalized medicine approach has a large effect on patient survival.[1] Approximately 50% of advanced adenocarcinomas have an oncogenic alteration, but only 20–25% of them are actionable oncogenic driver mutations.[2]

Epidermal growth factor receptor mutation

Epidermal growth factor receptor (*EGFR*) gene mutations are more frequent in Asian than Caucasian populations (~50% vs 10%), and more common in women and never-smokers. Mutations sensitive to EGFR tyrosine kinase inhibitors (TKI) are more frequently found in exon 19 (*deletion 19*) or in exon 21 (single point mutations, *L858R*).[3]

To date, nine randomized phase III trials have established reversible EGFR-TKI (erlotinib and gefitinib) and irreversible EGFR-TKI (afatinib) as standard first-line treatment in patients with NSCLC *EGFR* mutations. These agents have demonstrated improved response rates (RR) (56–84.6% vs 15–47.3%) and progression-free survival (PFS) (9.2–13.1 vs 4.6–6.9 months) compared with standard first-line platinum two-drug chemotherapy. To date, no differences in overall survival (OS) have been reported, possibly because of the high crossover rate.[4] Prospective data on afatinib use in uncommon *EGFR* mutations are available.[5]

A recent meta-analysis has reported that PFS with first-line EGFR-TKI compared with chemotherapy is greater in *Del19* than *L858R* (HR 0.24 vs 0.48).[6] However, there is no consensus about which inhibitor will maximize therapeutic efficacy in NSCLC patients with the *EGFR* mutation. Comparison of erlotinib and gefitinib did not show a significant difference in outcomes or toxicity between the two drugs.[7] A randomized phase IIb trial, which compared afatinib with gefitinib, showed a significant prolongation of PFS (11 vs 10.9 months, HR 0·73, 95%CI 0.57–0.95, p=0·0165) and overall RR (70.0% vs 56.0%, p=0.008) in favor of afatinib, independent of *EGFR* mutation subtype.[8] A phase III trial comparing dacomitinib with gefitinib is under way (ARCHER1050).

New strategies are needed to further improve PFS. Erlotinib plus bevacizumab improved median PFS compared with erlotinib (16 vs 9.7 months, HR 0.54, 95%CI 0.36–0.79, p=0.0015) in Asian patients.[9] In Caucasian patients, this strategy reported better outcome among T790M de novo-positive patients than T790M-negative patients (16 vs 10.5 months).[10]

After treatment with EGFR-TKI, tumors invariably develop acquired resistance (AR). Mechanisms of AR are secondary *EGFR* mutations, the bypassing of track signaling pathways or histological transformation.[11]

The gatekeeper T790M mutation in exon 20 of the *EGFR* gene is the most common type of AR mechanism observed in 49–63% of resistant biopsies.[11–13] Third-generation EGFR-TKIs osimertinib and rociletinib, which target both T790M and *EGFR*-sensitive mutations have been tested in phase I trials. Osimertinib has reported an RR of 61% and median PFS of 9.6 months in patients with T790M-positive NSCLC with AR to EGFR-TKI, and has been approved by the FDA.[14] Rociletinib has also reported an RR of 53% and PFS of 8 months in this population.[15] For those patients without T790M who develop AR, platinum-based chemotherapy seems to be a reasonable option beyond participating in clinical trials. The randomized phase III IMPRESS trial suggests that EGFR-TKI should be discontinued in patients with AR when commenced on two-drug second-line chemotherapy based on lack of PFS benefit and probable deleterious effect on OS.[16] For those patients with slow progressive disease, continuation of first-line EGFR-TKI beyond RECIST (response evaluation criteria in solid tumors) progression was possible for about another 3.9 months.[17] In cases of local progression, local therapies in conjunction with continued EGFR-TKI prolong survival.[18,19]

In two randomized phase III trials,[20,21] the efficacy of checkpoint inhibitors among patients with the *EGFR* mutation was lower than in the wild-type population, but dedicated clinical trials are ongoing to define the role of checkpoint inhibitors in this subgroup of patients.

Anaplastic lymphoma kinase gene rearrangement

ALK rearrangements (*ALK+*) result from inversions or translocations on chromosome 2 in about 5% of patients with NSCLC.[2] The gold-standard test for detecting *ALK* fusion is fluorescence in situ hybridization (FISH), using a cut-off point of 15% positive cells.[22] Immunohistochemistry (IHC) is also used as a diagnostic tool.

Crizotinib is a TKI that targets *ALK*, *ROS* and *MET* by competing for the binding pocket. It has been shown to improve PFS (7.7 vs 3.0 months) and RR (65% vs 20%) compared with pemetrexed or docetaxel as second-line treatment in *ALK+* patients.[23] It has also been shown to improve RR (74% vs 54%) and PFS (10.9 vs 7.0 months) compared with first-line platinum–pemetrexed combination chemotherapy in patients with *ALK+* NSCLC.[24] No benefit in OS was reported because of crossover.

The central nervous system (CNS) is the most common site of relapse or progression in patients taking crizotinib. A variety of mechanisms of AR to crizotinib have been identified,[25] among which new mutations in the *ALK* domain represent one-third of cases. Treatment at relapse may include local therapies while continuing crizotinib, or second-generation *ALK* inhibitors with higher potency and better penetrance of the CNS.

Ceritinib is approved by the US Food and Drug Administration (FDA) and the European Medicines Agency for the treatment of crizotinib-resistant patients. It has demonstrated clinical efficacy in patients with pretreated *ALK+* NSCLC (RR 56%, PFS 6.9 months) and in naive patients (RR 72%, PFS 18.4 months), even in patients with intracranial disease.[26]

Clinical data from a phase I/II trial investigating brigatinib (AP26113) in 78 patients with *ALK+* NSCLC pretreated with crizotinib, reported a RR of 71%, PFS of 13.4 months and 1-year OS of 100%.[27] On the basis of these results, the FDA has granted brigatinib a breakthrough-therapy designation for advanced *ALK+* NSCLC that has progressed to crizotinib. The ALTA-1L trial will compare brigatinib with crizotinib as first-line treatment.

Alectinib had a reponse rate of 48% in a phase II trial in patients pretreated with crizotinib,[28] with a median PFS of 8.9 months and clinical activity in patients with brain metastases (BM).[29] Based on these results, the FDA has approved alectinib in crizotinib-resistant patients. In crizotinib-naive patients, alectinib has demonstrated an RR of 94% and median PFS of 27 months.[30] The ongoing phase III AXEL trial is comparing alectinib with crizotinib in treatment-naive patients.

Lorlatinib (PF-06463922) is an *ALK/ROS1* inhibitor, which overcomes resistance to first- and second-generation *ALK* inhibitors and has high brain penetrance[31] with initial promising activity.

Other actionable alterations in NSCLC

BRAF mutations have been described in 2–4% of lung cancers, especially adenocarcinoma, with no ethnic or sex predominance. The V600E mutation accounts for 50% of cases.[32] Vemurafenib has demonstrated a response rate of 42% and median PFS of 7.3 months in a cohort of 20 patients with pretreated *BRAF* V600E NSCLC.[33] In a phase II study, dabrafenib demonstrated activity in patients with pretreated *BRAF* V600E mutation-positive NSCLC, with a RR of 32% and median PFS of 5.5 months.[34] Dabrafenib in combination with trametinib, a *MEK1* inhibitor, has demonstrated stronger activity (RR 63%) in the same population.[35]

ROS1 rearrangement occurs in 1–2% of NSCLC tumors; the FISH assay is the gold standard test,[36] with recent reports suggesting IHC as an alternative tool.[37] Crizotinib was tested in 50 patients with the *ROS1* rearrangement. The response rate was 72% with a median PFS of 19.2 months. In a European cohort of *ROS1* patients, crizotinib reported an 80% response rate and median PFS of 9.1 months.[38] Lorlatinib[31] and entrectinib[39] can overcome crizotinib resistance in *ROS1* tumors.

RET rearrangements occur in 1–2% of patients with NSCLC, especially in never smokers.[40] A small phase II study with cabozantinib reported a 44% response rate and median PFS of 7 months in 16 patients with *RET* fusions.[41] In mouse models, alectinib has reported activity in *RET*-rearranged NSCLC tumors.[42]

MET **amplification/mutation.** Aberrant overexpression, amplification and activating mutations of the MET receptor have been observed in specific subsets of lung tumors.[43] Crizotinib has shown clinical activity in high *MET*-amplified NSCLC.[44] In a French cohort of 18 patients with pretreated *MET*-amplified NSCLC, crizotinib had a RR of 39%.[45]

The oncogenic *MET* mutation in exon 14 occurs in 4% of lung adenocarcinomas,[46] especially in older women (~75 years),[47] and it confers clinical sensitivity to MET inhibitors[48] such as crizotinib and cabozantinib.[46]

HER2 **mutations** occur in about 2% of lung adenocarcinomas.[49] In a European cohort of 101 patients with *HER2* exon-20 insertion NSCLC, *HER2* therapies achieved a 50.9% RR and median PFS of 4.8 months.[50] Dacomitinib has also demonstrated activity in this population (12% RR in patients with *HER2* mutations vs 0% in *HER2*-amplified patients, with median OS of 9 months in the *HER2*-mutant subgroup).[51]

NTRK1 **and** *NTRK2* **rearrangements** occur in 1–2% of patients with NSCLC. Entrectinib has had promising results in this subpopulation of lung cancer patients.[39]

Key points – personalized treatment in advanced NSCLC

- All patients with adenocarcinoma should have mutation testing for *EGFR* and *ALK-MET* at diagnosis.
- *EGFR* mutations at any stage should have treatment with a tyrosine kinase inhibitor until symptomatic progression.
- Patients with *ALK-MET* or *ROS1* translocations respond well to crizotinib.
- Second-generation drugs are becoming available.
- Other driver mutations and targeted therapies need acceleration into the clinic for patient benefit.

References

1. Kris MG, Johnson BE, Berry LD et al. Using multiplexed assays of oncogenic drivers in lung cancers to select targeted drugs. *JAMA* 2014;311:1998–2006.

2. Barlesi F, Mazieres J, Merlio JP et al. Routine molecular profiling of patients with advanced non-small-cell lung cancer: results of a 1-year nationwide programme of the French Cooperative Thoracic Intergroup (IFCT). *Lancet* 2016;387:1415–26.

3. Gahr S, Stoehr R, Geissinger E et al. *EGFR* mutational status in a large series of Caucasian European NSCLC patients: data from daily practice. *Br J Cancer* 2013;109: 1821–8.

4. Reguart N, Remon J. Common *EGFR*-mutated subgroups (Del19/ L858R) in advanced non-small-cell lung cancer: chasing better outcomes with tyrosine kinase inhibitors. *Future Oncol* 2015;11:1245–57.

5. Yang JC, Sequist LV, Geater SL et al. Clinical activity of afatinib in patients with advanced non-small-cell lung cancer harbouring uncommon *EGFR* mutations: a combined post-hoc analysis of LUX-Lung 2, LUX-Lung 3, and LUX-Lung 6. *Lancet Oncol* 2015;16:830–8.

6. Lee CK, Wu Y-L, Ding PN et al. Impact of specific epidermal growth factor receptor (*EGFR*) mutations and clinical characteristics on outcomes after treatment with EGFR tyrosine kinase inhibitors versus chemotherapy in *EGFR*-mutant lung cancer: a meta-analysis. *J Clin Oncol* 2015;33:1958–65.

7. Yang JJ, Zhou Q, Yan HH et al. A randomized controlled trial of erlotinib versus gefitinib in advanced non-small-cell lung cancer harboring *EGFR* mutations (CTONG0901). *J Thorac Oncol* 2015;10:S321.

8. Park K, Tan E, Zhang L et al. Afatinib (A) vs gefitinib (G) as first-line treatment for patients (pts) with advanced non-small cell lung cancer (NSCLC) harboring activating *EGFR* mutations: results of the global, randomized, open-label, Phase IIb trial LUX-Lung 7 (LL7). *Ann Oncol* 2015;26(suppl 9):161–2.

9. Seto T, Kato T, Nishio M et al. Erlotinib alone or with bevacizumab as first-line therapy in patients with advanced non-squamous non-small-cell lung cancer harbouring *EGFR* mutations (JO25567): an open-label, randomised, multicentre, phase 2 study. *Lancet Oncol* 2014;15:1236–44.

10. Stahel R, Dafni U, Gautschi O et al. A phase II trial of erlotinib (E) and bevacizumab (B) in patients with advanced non-small-cell lung cancer with activating epidermal growth factor receptor (*EGFR*) mutations with and without T790M mutation. Spanish Lung Cancer Group (SLCG) and the European Thoracic Oncology Platform (ETOP) BELIEF trial. European Cancer Congress. Abstract 3BA. Presented September 28, 2015.

11. Sequist LV, Waltman BA, Dias-Santagata D et al. Genotypic and histological evolution of lung cancers acquiring resistance to EGFR inhibitors. *Sci Transl Med* 2011;3:75ra26.

12. Arcila ME, Oxnard GR, Nafa K et al. Rebiopsy of lung cancer patients with acquired resistance to EGFR inhibitors and enhanced detection of the T790M mutation using a locked nucleic acid-based assay. *Clin Cancer Res* 2011;17:1169–80.

13. Yu HA, Arcila ME, Rekhtman N et al. Analysis of tumor specimens at the time of acquired resistance to EGFR TKI therapy in 155 patients with *EGFR*-mutant lung cancers. *Clin Cancer Res* 2013;19:2240–7.

14. Jänne PA, Yang JC-H, Kim D-W et al. AZD9291 in EGFR inhibitor-resistant non-small-cell lung cancer. *N Engl J Med* 2015;372:1689–99.

15. Sequist LV, Goldman JW, Wakelee HA et al. Efficacy of rociletinib (CO-1686) in plasma-genotyped T790M-positive non-small cell lung cancer (NSCLC) patients (pts). *J Clin Oncol* 2015;33(suppl; abstr 8001).

16. Soria JC, Wu YL, Nakagawa K et al. Gefitinib plus chemotherapy versus placebo plus chemotherapy in *EGFR*-mutation-positive non-small-cell lung cancer after progression on first-line gefitinib (IMPRESS): a phase 3 randomised trial. *Lancet Oncol* 2015;16:990–8.

17. Park K, Yu CJ, Kim SW et al. First-line erlotinib therapy until and beyond response evaluation criteria in solid tumors progression in Asian patients with epidermal growth factor receptor mutation-positive non-small-cell lung cancer: the ASPIRATION study. *JAMA Oncol* 2016;2:305–12.

18. Weickhardt AJ, Scheier B, Burke JM et al. Local ablative therapy of oligoprogressive disease prolongs disease control by tyrosine kinase inhibitors in oncogene addicted non-small cell lung cancer. *J Thorac Oncol* 2012;7:1807–14.

19. Yu HA, Sima CS, Huang J et al. Local therapy with continued EGFR tyrosine kinase inhibitor therapy as a treatment strategy in *EGFR* mutant advanced lung cancers that have developed acquired resistance to EGFR tyrosine kinase inhibitors. *J Thorac Oncol* 2013;8:346–51.

20. Borghaei H, Paz-Ares L, Horn L et al. Nivolumab versus docetaxel in advanced nonsquamous non-small-cell lung cancer. *N Engl J Med* 2015;373:1627–39.

21. Herbst RS, Baas P, Kim DW et al. Pembrolizumab versus docetaxel for previously treated, PD-L1-positive, advanced non-small-cell lung cancer (KEYNOTE-010): a randomised controlled trial. *Lancet* 2016;387:1540–50.

22. Kwak EL, Bang Y-J, Camidge DR et al. Anaplastic lymphoma kinase inhibition in non-small-cell lung cancer. *N Engl J Med* 2010;363:1693–703.

23. Shaw AT, Kim D-W, Nakagawa K et al. Crizotinib versus chemotherapy in advanced *ALK*-positive lung cancer. *N Engl J Med* 2013;368:2385–94.

24. Solomon BJ, Mok T, Kim D-W et al. First-line crizotinib versus chemotherapy in *ALK*-positive lung cancer. *N Engl J Med* 2014;371:2167–77.

25. Doebele RC, Pilling AB, Aisner DL et al. Mechanisms of resistance to crizotinib in patients with *ALK* gene rearranged non-small cell lung cancer. *Clin Cancer Res* 2012;18: 1472–82.

26. Kim DW, Mehra R, Tan DS et al. Activity and safety of ceritinib in patients with *ALK*-rearranged non-small-cell lung cancer (ASCEND-1): updated results from the multicentre, open-label, phase 1 trial. *Lancet Oncol* 2016;17:452–63.

27. Camidge DR, Bazhenova LA, Salgia R et al. Safety and efficacy of brigatinib (AP26113) in advanced malignancies, including *ALK+* non-small cell lung cancer. *J Clin Oncol* 2015;33(suppl; abstr 8062).

28. Shaw AT, Gandhi L, Gadgeel S et al. Alectinib in *ALK*-positive, crizotinib-resistant, non-small-cell lung cancer: a single-group, multicentre, phase 2 trial, *Lancet Oncol* 2016;17:234–42.

29. Ou S-HI, Ahn JS, De Petris L et al. Alectinib in crizotinib-refractory *ALK*-rearranged non-small-cell lung cancer: a phase II global study. *J Clin Oncol* 2016;34:661–8.

30. Seto T, Kiura K, Nishio M et al. CH5424802 (RO5424802) for patients with *ALK*-rearranged advanced non-small-cell lung cancer (AF-001JP study): a single-arm, open-label, phase 1-2 study, *Lancet Oncol* 2013;14:590–8.

31. Zou HY, Friboulet L, Kodack DP et al. PF-06463922, an *ALK/ROS1* inhibitor, overcomes resistance to first and second generation *ALK* inhibitors in preclinical models. *Cancer Cell* 2015;28:70–81.

32. Nguyen-Ngoc T, Bouchaab H, Adjei AA, Peters S. *BRAF* alterations as therapeutic targets in non-small-cell lung cancer. *J Thorac Oncol* 2015;10:1396–403.

33. Hyman DM, Puzanov I, Subbiah V et al. Vemurafenib in multiple nonmelanoma cancers with *BRAF* V600 mutations. *N Engl J Med* 2015;373:726–36.

34. Planchard D, Mazieres J, Riely GJ et al. Interim results of phase II study BRF113928 of dabrafenib in *BRAF* V600E mutation-positive non-small cell lung cancer (NSCLC) patients. *J Clin Oncol* 2013; 31(suppl; abstr 8009).

35. Planchard D, Groen HJM, Kim TM et al. Interim results of a phase II study of the BRAF inhibitor (BRAFi) dabrafenib (D) in combination with the *MEK* inhibitor trametinib (T) in patients (pts) with *BRAF* V600E mutated (mut) metastatic non-small cell lung cancer (NSCLC). *J Clin Oncol* 2015;33(suppl; abstr 8006).

36. Shaw AT, Ou S-HI, Bang Y-J et al. Crizotinib in *ROS1*-rearranged non-small-cell lung cancer. *N Engl J Med* 2014;371:1963–71.

37. Boyle TA, Masago K, Ellison KE et al. *ROS1* immunohistochemistry among major genotypes of non-small-cell lung cancer. *Clin Lung Cancer* 2015;16:106–11.

38. Mazières J, Zalcman G, Crinò L et al. Crizotinib therapy for advanced lung adenocarcinoma and a *ROS1* rearrangement: results from the EUROS1 cohort. *J Clin Oncol* 2015;33:992–9.

39. Ardini E, Menichincheri M, Banfi P et al. Entrectinib, a *Pan-TRK, ROS1* and *ALK* inhibitor with activity in multiple molecularly defined cancer indications. *Mol Cancer Ther* 2016;15:628–39.

40. Michels S, Scheel AH, Scheffler M et al. Clinicopathological characteristics of *RET* rearranged lung cancer in European patients. *J Thorac Oncol* 2016;11:122–7.

41. Drilon AE, Sima CS, Somwar R et al. Phase II study of cabozantinib for patients with advanced *RET*-rearranged lung cancers. *J Clin Oncol* 2015;33(suppl; abstr 8007).

42. Kodama T, Tsukaguchi T, Satoh Y et al. Alectinib shows potent antitumor activity against *RET*-rearranged non-small cell lung cancer, *Mol Cancer Ther* 2014;13:2910–18.

43. Sadiq AA, Salgia R. *MET* as a possible target for non-small-cell lung cancer. *J Clin Oncol* 2013;31:1089–96.

44. Camidge DR, Ou S-HI, Shapiro G et al. Efficacy and safety of crizotinib in patients with advanced c-*MET*-amplified non-small cell lung cancer (NSCLC). *J Clin Oncol* 2014;32(suppl; abstr 8001).

45. Hamard C, Ruppert AM, Lavole A et al. News about targeted therapies in non-small-cell lung cancer in 2015 (except immuno-therapy). *Ann Pathol* 2016;36:63–72.

46. Paik PK, Drilon A, Fan P-D et al. Response to *MET* inhibitors in patients with stage IV lung adenocarcinomas harboring *MET* mutations causing exon 14 skipping. *Cancer Discov* 2015;5:842–9.

47. Awad MM, Oxnard GR, Jackman DM et al. *MET* exon 14 mutations in non-small-cell lung cancer are associated with advanced age and stage-dependent *MET* genomic amplification and c-Met overexpression. *J Clin Oncol* 2016;34:721–30.

48. Frampton GM, Ali SM, Rosenzweig M et al. Activation of *MET* via diverse exon 14 splicing alterations occurs in multiple tumor types and confers clinical sensitivity to MET inhibitors, *Cancer Discov* 2015;5:850–9.

49. Mazières J, Peters S, Lepage B et al. Lung cancer that harbors an *HER2* mutation: epidemiologic characteristics and therapeutic perspectives. *J Clin Oncol* 2013;31:1997–2003.

50. Mazières J, Barlesi F, Filleron T et al. Lung cancer patients with *HER2* mutations treated with chemotherapy and *HER2*-targeted drugs: results from the European EUHER2 cohort. *Ann Oncol* 2016;27:281–6.

51. Kris MG, Camidge DR, Giaccone G et al. Targeting *HER2* aberrations as actionable drivers in lung cancers: phase II trial of the pan-*HER* tyrosine kinase inhibitor dacomitinib in patients with *HER2*-mutant or amplified tumors. *Ann Oncol* 2015;26:1421–7.

Useful resources

UK

British Lung Foundation
Helpline: 03000 030 555
Tel: +44 (0)20 7688 5555
blf.org.uk

British Thoracic Society
Tel: +44 (0)20 7831 8778
bts@brit-thoracic.org.uk
brit-thoracic.org.uk

Cancer Research UK
Tel: +44 (0)30 0123 1022
cancerresearchuk.org

Macmillan Cancer Support
Toll-free: 0808 808 00 00
Tel: +44 (0)20 7840 7841
macmillan.org.uk

Roy Castle Lung Cancer
Foundation
Tel: 0333 323 7200
roycastle.org

UK Lung Cancer Screening Trial
ukls.org

UK Lung Cancer Coalition
Tel: +44 (0)1675 477605
info@uklcc.org.uk
uklcc.org.uk

USA

American Cancer Society
Toll-free: 1 800 227 2345
cancer.org

American Lung Association
Toll-free: 1 800 586 4872
lung.org

Lung Cancer Foundation of
America
lcfamerica.org

lungcancer.org (CancerCare®)
Toll-free: 1 800 813 4673
Tel: +1 212 712 8400
info@cancercare.org
lungcancer.org

Lung Cancer Research Foundation
Tel: +1 212 588 1580
info@lungfund.org
lungcancerresearchfoundation.org

National Cancer Institute
Toll-free: 1 800 422 6237
cancer.gov

International

Cancer Association of South Africa
Toll-free: 0800 22 66 22
Tel: +27 (0)11 616 7662
info@cansa.org.za
cansa.org.za

European Lung Foundation
Tel: +44 (0)114 267 2875
info@europeanlung.org
europeanlung.org

European Respiratory Society
Tel: +41 21 213 01 01
ersnet.org

International Association for the Study of Lung Cancer
Tel: 1 855 464 2752
iaslc.org

The Lung Association (Canada)
Ask an expert: 1 866 717 2673
Toll-free: 1 888 566 5864
lung.ca

Lung Cancer Canada
Toll-free: 1 888 445 4403
Tel: +1 416 785 3439
info@lungcancercanada.ca
lungcancercanada.ca

Lung Cancer (Cancer Australia)
Toll-free: 1 800 624 973
Tel: +61 (0)2 9357 9400
lung-cancer.canceraustralia.gov.au

Lung Cancer Europe
luce@etop-eu.org
lungcancereurope.eu

Lung Foundation Australia
Toll-free: 1 800 654 301
lungfoundation.com.au

FastTest

You've read the book ... now test yourself with key questions from the authors

- Go to the FastTest for this title
  FREE at fastfacts.com
- Approximate time **10 minutes**
- For best retention of the key issues, try taking the FastTest before and after reading

Index

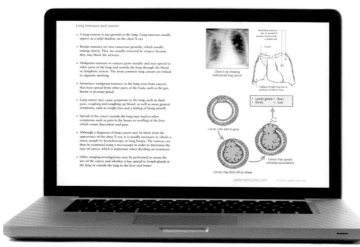

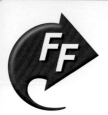

Fast Facts – the ultimate medical handbook series covers over 60 topics, including:

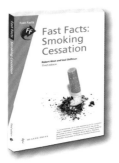

Fast Facts:
Smoking
Cessation

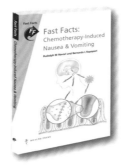

Fast Facts:
Chemotherapy-Induced
Nausea & Vomiting

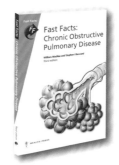

Fast Facts:
Chronic Obstructive
Pulmonary Disease

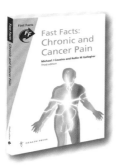

Fast Facts:
Chronic and
Cancer Pain

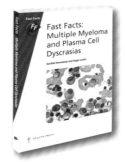

Fast Facts:
Multiple Myeloma
and Plasma Cell
Dyscrasias

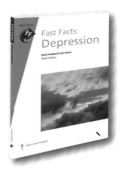

Fast Facts:
Depression

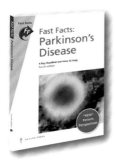

Fast Facts:
Parkinson's
Disease

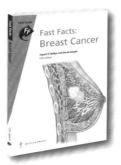

Fast Facts:
Breast Cancer

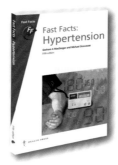

Fast Facts:
Hypertension

fastfacts.com

Our hope is that this Fast Facts *title helps you to improve your practice and, in turn, improves the health of your patients*

What will you do next?

Use this space to write some action points that have come from reading this book and testing yourself. And don't worry if you pass this on to a colleague, senior or junior; they are bound to find them interesting and may wish to add their own.

Action Point 1

Action Point 2

Action Point 3

If you have the time to share them with us, or you have suggestions of how to improve the next edition, we'd love to hear from you at
feedback@fastfacts.com